Raised by her grandmother in outback New South Wales, Sonya Melbourne is the only child of a mentally ill mother and criminal father. Her first-hand experience of childhood in an environment of poverty, illness and dysfunction has led Sonya to want to share inspirational stories of hope.

In her late teens, she was employed as a community aid worker with a local council home assistance scheme, where she assisted ill and disadvantaged members of the community in their own homes. She went on to build a successful career as a global human resource executive.

In 2006, Sonya became Managing Director of the Brisbane-based human resource and management consulting group, Astor Levin Pty Ltd.

Sonya lives in Brisbane with her husband Colin. They have two grown daughters and two granddaughters.

An accomplished writer, Sonya's business-related articles are regularly published in trade magazines. *Inspired Recovery* is her first book.

For
My husband Colin – the love of my life
Mum – loving, resilient and courageous – my inspiration
My two beautiful daughters, Nicholle and Kahlea, who have brought such
love, laughter and sunshine to my world
My wonderful sons-in-law, Andrew and Alex
and my delicious grandchildren.

INSPIRED RECOVERY

True stories of hope and
recovery from mental illness

as told to

SONYA MELBOURNE

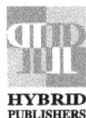

HYBRID
PUBLISHERS

Published by Hybrid Publishers
Melbourne Victoria Australia

First published 2010

National Library of Australia Cataloguing-in-Publication entry:
Author: Melbourne, Sonya.
Title: Inspired recovery / Sonya Melbourne.

ISBN: 9781921665011 (pbk.)

Subjects: Ex-mental patients – Australia – Biography.
Mental illness – Australia – Biography.
Mentally ill – Australia – Biography.

Dewey Number: 616.89092

Cover design: Tali Foster-Snowdon, JSA Design
Printed in Australia by McPherson's Printing Group

Foreword

If you need to be reminded about the resilience of the human spirit, please read *Inspired Recovery*.

Each chapter provides a glimpse into a remarkable and courageous journey. It is a great privilege to read these narratives, sincere and full of wisdom. They describe how people cope in the face of psychological stress and serious mental illness. Alas, they also bring into sharp relief how much more work needs to be done in order to help people stay on their individual pathways to recovery.

Historians tell us that the compassion and strength of a society can be judged on how that society treats their minority groups. The true stories told in this book about how we help people recover from mental illness suggest that our society still has a long way to go.

Ignorance breeds stigma. This book will help reduce some of this ignorance.

The book also provides templates for others struggling to cope with mental illness – here are tried and true suggestions, based on lived experience. Not all of these suggestions will work for all individuals – we need much more research into the causes of, and optimal treatments for, mental illness – but this book is tonic for the spirit and will inspire many more along the road to recovery.

Professor John McGrath AM, MD, PhD
Queensland Centre for Mental Health Research

Contents

Acknowledgments and thanks

Sincere gratitude to each of the contributors. I remain in awe of your personal courage and resilience. Choosing to share your experiences in this way has enriched my life and will no doubt give hope to thousands of people in need. This is your book – well done!

Sincere thanks to Anna Rosner Blay, a remarkably talented writer and Managing Editor at Hybrid Publishers. Your support and belief in this book and its message has brought it to life. Thank you.

Thanks also to the charitable organisations who work tirelessly to support those among us that need help. Your work is a blessing to all of society.

I am truly grateful to freelance editor, Deborah Brodie. Your advice and encouragement have been appreciated every bit as much as your expertise, talent and professionalism. My appreciation also to Eddie Retelj and Margaret Johnson. Your suggestions and guidance were nothing short of wonderful.

Thanks also to Kahlea Brown, my writing assistant. A talented young writer herself, Kahlea's help in organising, transcribing, proofreading and the myriad of other essential tasks was absolutely priceless. You joined me on this journey, Kahlea, and it would not have been the same without you.

Above all, I humbly express gratitude to the Universe and to God, through whom all things are possible.

Preface

My mother's mental illnesses shaped my early life.

She suffers bipolar disorder, schizoaffective disorder, borderline personality disorder and generalised anxiety disorder. She also has a number of serious physical ailments and has suffered horrific physical and emotional abuse throughout her life.

An only child, I was bullied by neighbourhood kids for being 'the zombie's daughter' or 'the psycho's kid who must be a psycho too'. I was laughed at, threatened, chased, abused, and on one occasion even spat on (memorable!). But these experiences were fleeting. Watching my mother suffer and being unable to help her was the real challenge. It took me many years to accept this.

Witnessing her grow as a person while retaining her gentle nature, despite all the odds, has humbled me. And she is not the only one among us with such fearlessness and strength.

The stories you are about to read are not accounts of mental illness. These powerful true accounts explore the journeys of fellow human beings who, among other aspects of their life, manage mental illness.

They welcome us into their experience with courage and honesty. They willingly share their pain and also their joy, in the hope that we will begin to understand; in the hope that tomorrow will feel a little brighter for us, so that we can always know that there is a way through.

There is hope.

Sonya Melbourne

Note: Real names have been used throughout except for the pseudonyms Scarlett, Ciara and Imogen, chosen by the contributors themselves.

One: Maree

My father called me the *miracle baby* after I survived my mother's attempt to abort me, with a knitting needle, in an uncle's backyard. The ninth of twelve children born to alcoholic parents, I arrived three months premature. I weighed only one kilogram at birth and was not expected to live, so an immediate baptism was arranged. Once it was clear that I would survive, my mother decided that she didn't want me, and I was never taken home to be with my siblings.

At eight months old I was placed in my first foster home. I was removed from this placement when it was discovered that I had been mistreated. Custody was legally awarded to the Department of Child Welfare and I became a ward of the State. By this time each of my siblings had also become wards of the State, due to our parents' neglect and incompetent guardianship.

At the age of two, I was placed with my fourth and final placement, a foster family in Sydney. Unfortunately, my placement with this 'respectable' Catholic couple and four of their natural children marked the beginning of the worst sixteen years of my life. Despite this, I considered my foster parents as my parents, and I still do.

My father often told me that I was his favourite girl. He was the only person who played with me, showed affection and gave me praise. In turn, I idolised him and felt he could do no wrong. My mother, on the other hand, was openly hostile towards me. She was a strict Catholic who ruled myself and her other foster child, Wayne, with an iron fist. My mother was in charge of discipline while my father took a passive 'benevolent-but-helpless-parent' role.

The contrast between my mother's hostility and my father's goodwill provided fertile ground for me to develop an unrealistic, idealised view of my father. I absolutely adored him. I found solace in his attention, even as he sexually abused me.

In order to maintain the fantasy of being loved by at least one member of my family, I tried to justify his abuse as a sign of his inner pain and suffering, caused by my horrible mother. I could not disclose details of my life to anyone, as I lived in fear of being not only directly punished, but more importantly, expelled from the family. This was an eventuality that I was prepared to pay any price to avoid. I was told that if I ever misbehaved, I would be sent away to the *Home for Bad Girls*. This threat alone was terrifying enough to keep me in line most of the time. Nonetheless, I was beaten by my mother almost every Sunday after church, if I committed any misdemeanour such as taking my hat off, standing when I should have knelt, fidgeting or not sitting still. So, I grew up believing I was bad. I also became completely compliant. I learned that 'love' was conditional on accepting abuse in order to receive whatever crumbs of kindness might be given from time to time. It wasn't until many years later I was able to see the difference between love and abuse, and to identify sexual abuse as *abuse*.

The sexual abuse continued long into my adolescence. My father often came into the bathroom while I was bathing, to shave my arms, legs, and bikini line with a razor. He would tell me that my mother had asked him to do so. This confused me deeply. If she wanted him to do that, what would she think of the sexual abuse? Did she know? I wasn't sure. I once hinted to a friend's mother that my father 'did things' to me and that I was unhappy at home. The news came straight back to my mother, who administered a severe beating, knocked me to the ground and screamed, 'Whatever happens in this family stays in the family!'

When I was at my lowest ebb, I would go out onto the back concrete step of my parents' house and look up at the stars. I believed the stars were 'holes in the floorboards of heaven'. For long periods I stared up at those stars, trying to figure a way to die and 'slip away' quietly. I was eleven years old.

The stress of my home environment prevented me from performing to the extent of my capability in school. I was often depressed, which made it difficult to concentrate for any period of time. I was unable to take in information and, if I did, I struggled to retain it. I sat at the back of the classroom and spent my time daydreaming about death or staring into space. Other times I took the role of class clown. My moods became unstable. One minute I would feel happy, the next I would be in a raging temper.

School seemed unreal and somewhat irrelevant to me. Because I didn't fit in, I became defiant and rebellious. On one occasion, my mother was called up to the school to discuss my rebellious behaviour. She found this a humiliating experience, so I received a brutal assault that afternoon when I arrived home.

I was constantly taunted and criticised by my mother. She seemed to delight in telling me I was *dumb, stupid and slow,* and that I would *never amount to anything.* These daily messages, along with the assaults, confirmed my belief that I was powerless to improve my situation. For years I believed that I was indeed stupid and that any further studies were out of the question.

I was thirteen years old when I found out that I was a foster child and these weren't my biological parents. A friend at school told me one day during our lunch break. I was initially confused and wondered why my friend would create such a story. That night I confronted my mother, who confirmed this was, in fact, the truth. Things suddenly made sense. I finally understood why a District Officer came to our home on a regular basis. I could always tell if he was due for a visit, as my mother went out of her way to be kind to me.

It was also around this time that my brother-in-law began sexually assaulting me. My sister's wedding brought out the family dysfunction on all fronts. Two weeks after my sister returned from her honeymoon, I was left alone in their new home with my brother-in-law while wedding presents were collected from my parents' home. My sister was totally unaware that her husband raped me that day. After the assault, once everyone had returned to the house, the family ate lunch together. No one asked why I was particularly quiet and unwilling to eat.

The sexual abuse from my father finally ended when I left home at the age of eighteen, following a huge family fight. The conflict initially erupted between my parents and my foster brother, Wayne. Since Wayne had joined the family unit, my mother had been constantly telling him he would end up in jail and that he was a no-hoper. After years of having this message repeatedly drummed into his head, the inevitable happened and he committed a crime. Wayne stole a bike but became stranded following a flat tyre. My parents refused to assist him, and when he arrived home he was ordered to leave the family home. I adored Wayne, so I stood up for him. I, too, was told to leave.

As I packed my bags, I noticed that my father did nothing to contradict my mother's edict. I was angry that he continued to allow her to take control, without challenging her or supporting me. As my father stood at the doorway of my bedroom, I told him that I would never forget what he had done to me. I left and never returned.

I sank into a deep depression. I became withdrawn, fearful and self-destructive, and lived a negative lifestyle, albeit with a new-found freedom. I met young people my own age at parties, discos and pubs; people who were willing to supply me with drugs. In order to remain sane, drugs became my great escape.

There was nothing I wouldn't try in order to get high. On drugs, I felt that I could be anyone I wanted to be. I had a driving need to punish myself, so when I was involved in a motor vehicle accident that left me with chronic pain, it was easy to become addicted to prescription painkillers to maintain a numb state of mind.

I smoked liberal quantities of marijuana. I also dabbled in heroin, but I couldn't stand the sight of a needle, so a junkie friend put the needle in my arm. On two occasions I had a serious physical reaction to the heroin and was rushed to hospital, each time discharging myself while still sick. I decided to abandon heroin and started doing the rounds of doctors' surgeries to source multiple prescriptions for pain medication.

I took twice as many drugs as others around me, and I couldn't have cared less about the effect they had. I didn't care if they killed me. I had a greater love/trust relationship with drugs than I had ever experienced with my foster family.

I also consumed huge amounts of alcohol, but I found that it didn't provide the same buoyant effect as other drugs. Alcohol enabled me to express my anger, rage and feelings of hostility, and even enabled me to cry. I often wondered what I had done wrong to deserve what I got.

When intoxicated, I could tolerate a high level of physical pain, so I would cut parts of my body. When drinking heavily, I kept company with abusive and aggressive people; previously I had spent time with accepting and submissive drug users. At the end of the day, neither drugs nor alcohol gave me what I was searching for. They simply gave me a way to cope at that time.

Over the years, for absolutely no apparent reason, I often went out of control. My mood suddenly shifted and the most trivial thing would irritate or agitate me. My reaction to situations or events was disproportionate and extreme. I would fly into quick sudden rages at anything or anyone. If I pressed the wrong button on the stereo, I smashed it. If I couldn't get others to understand my way of thinking, I was argumentative. When I couldn't do a simple task, I smashed a window or broke the nearest item available. I was easily irritated, often for no reason. There were times when I experienced highly irrational thoughts and hallucinations. I didn't understand what was happening to me. I would take on any dare and accept extraordinary risks. The thoughts and threat to kill myself were very real and constantly at the back of my mind. When these subsided, I would again become cheerful, bright and funny – until the roller coaster ride began all over again.

After I left home, my brother-in-law continued to sexually assault me. I felt low about myself and very confused. I endured my brother-in-law's performances through a drug haze or drunkenness, with his active encouragement. He was potentially dangerous and threatened me never to tell what was happening, for fear of retribution. He told me clearly that if I reported what had gone on, some sort of 'accident' would happen to me.

As a result of my brother-in-law's assaults, I became pregnant. As soon as I discovered this, I became absolutely determined to give my baby the best start in life. I stopped all drug and alcohol use immediately and ate as well as I could afford to, for the sake of my unborn child. In 1978 I gave birth to a baby girl, and my brother-in-law dropped out of my life completely, wanting to have no involvement with the pregnancy or the child.

I soon realised that I was in no position to care for myself or the baby, so I surrendered my infant for adoption. I started moving from place to place, suburb to suburb and job to job. Once my infant had been adopted, my brother-in-law put a lot of pressure on me to resume the practice of servicing his sexual needs. By this time, compliance and learned helplessness were deeply ingrained within me and I felt that I had no option. I also returned to my drug and alcohol habits.

I was deeply grief-stricken at the loss of my child. Friends were concerned for me and, although I was reluctant to see a doctor, I eventually did so and was referred to a psychiatrist. I had never seen a psychiatrist before, so I didn't know what to expect. Unfortunately, this psychiatrist showed absolutely no interest in anything I had to say. He seemed almost bored. He made no eye contact and was not ready, willing or able to become part of the process. Talking to him was like releasing a message into space. I felt uneasy, uncomfortable and unimportant. Then something inside me suddenly became undone. I had a major meltdown. I yelled, screamed and literally threw his fee in his face. I stormed out to reception and swore I would never come back.

At the age of 24, I began to search for my biological family, and found three of them that same year. I learned that my biological mother suffered from depression and my biological father suffered from schizophrenia. I met my siblings over the next nine years.

The reunion with my biological family was no fairytale. One of my biological brothers took his life at the age of thirty, after a period of depression. Another of my biological brothers, who also suffered from depression, had died at the age of 26 after falling from the roof of a building. We don't know if the fall was accidental or deliberate.

In October 1981, after three drug overdoses, I finally entered a residential Therapeutic Drug and Alcohol Rehabilitation Centre. I was blackmailed into entering the program by a friend who threatened to have me arrested for my drug taking if I did not voluntarily seek treatment. While in the centre, I behaved in a rebellious manner and refused to cooperate in any way. The drug rehab program gave me the provisional diagnosis of bipolar disorder which, at the time, required me to take Lithium. I refused the treatment, the medication and the blood tests. I discharged myself from the program three times over a period of two years, before finally following it through to completion.

Three years later, near the end of the program, I suffered a severe psychotic episode. I began to hallucinate and self-mutilate. I was rushed to the acute psychiatric care unit of a major hospital. I was thirty years old, and this was my first admission to a psychiatric unit. I wasn't really aware of where I was at the time, as I had lost touch with reality.

No one knew of my world. Physically, I didn't look or feel any different than I always had, but emotionally I felt numb. This place was like no other place and the people were like none I had ever met.

I was scared. I saw a female patient bashing her head against a glass window as she was sitting on a chair, yelling obscenities. It was at this point that I first had a glimpse of where I was, but I felt I didn't really exist. It felt as if I was in an alien world: a place that I had sworn never to enter, no matter what. I didn't want to be like my family.

After initially demonstrating strong resistance to being in the ward, I started testing staff to the limits, in an effort to establish whether or not I could trust them. After three months, my primary therapist, Marie-Pierre, a psychiatric social worker, ascertained that I was suffering from post-traumatic stress disorder. For the first time in my life, I felt that I was not being blamed or made to feel defective for how I was. My past experiences were recognised as being the core of my 'condition'. There was a reason for me being the way I was!

As my primary therapist changed jobs over the years, I transferred to wherever she was, and eventually I went with her into private practice. Marie-Pierre took me under her wing and worked with me for many years. She helped me deal with many issues from my past as well as everyday issues I faced. Over the years we often had a battle of wits and the ride was rough. But together we went through it all – the thunder, the storms and dark windy days. Together we examined every facet of how abuse had affected my life. I learned new ways of dealing with the effects of my past and started finding reasons to live.

I came from a position of having no home of my own, no career, no friends, no caring family, and I had just begun to adopt a drug-free lifestyle for the first time in many years. I had a big task ahead of me.

In one particular session, Marie-Pierre challenged my poor behaviour and unpredictable mood swings and issued an ultimatum. She insisted I go to my doctor and get a referral to see a psychiatrist or she simply would not work with me any more. I argued and resisted to no avail. She was adamant, so I complied. I visited a psychiatrist and, in 1996, was given the definitive diagnosis of bipolar affective disorder with complex post-traumatic stress disorder. It was necessary for me to go on medication, and this time I complied. Although I was devastated, I returned to Marie-Pierre and my therapy continued.

In 1988 I had begun working with Kids in Care and was offered the opportunity to undertake a study skills program. I went on to successfully complete the Associate Diploma in Youth Work at TAFE. I had unearthed a thirst for knowledge. In 1993, I applied as a mature-age student to enter an undergraduate university degree in welfare studies, and was accepted!

This was a busy time, filled with therapy, work and study. I decided, with Marie-Pierre's support, to contact the police and report the abuse I had suffered. Finally, in June 1996, I completed statements regarding my assailants. I was so traumatised it took me three months to complete them.

My moods continued to fluctuate, and I cycled in and out of a depressed state. When I am in extreme states of panic, agitation, suicidal or self-destructive moods, it is imperative that I have access to a safe holding-environment. This has necessitated admission to psychiatric hospitals. Unfortunately, during some of my admissions to hospital, I have witnessed, and been subject to, poor treatment. In one particular psychiatric hospital, I was taunted by a male psychiatric nurse and challenged to throw my bread-and-butter knife at him during my meal. I took on his dare, aimed and threw. Within seconds my chair was kicked from under me and I was thrown backwards onto the floor. I was restrained and given an injection. Despite all my attempts to explain the situation, no one would listen. I was too unwell to recognise the 'set up' or the consequences and I remained in a daze for the rest of that day.

During this same admission, I slipped out of the ward one night with two other patients, unnoticed. We caught a taxi at the front of the hospital and went to the local Pizza Hut Restaurant. We ventured back into the ward two hours later. None of the staff had even noticed our absence.

I have observed a certain 'culture' among the staff of some public psychiatric hospitals. They do not like to be disturbed. Quite often they can be seen in the office reading the paper or a magazine, chatting to each other or spending time doing other things, rather than responding to a patient who needs their assistance, and who is knocking on the staff door. I witnessed, first hand, a young woman in distress who approached staff repeatedly. Each time she was told to come back in ten minutes, they would come to get her or they'd be with her shortly. Every excuse was given and 'shortly' became an eternity. In what I can only imagine as sheer desperation, this young woman threw herself out of the second-floor lounge-room window that afternoon, and died on the pavement below. It all happened very quickly. The staff finally came out of the office, but it was too late.

There was no debriefing for patients. I remember closing my eyes to sleep that night with the vision of her charging towards the window and going straight through it.

On another of my early hospital admissions, a fellow patient set herself on fire in the female toilet. The smell of burning flesh will remain with me for the rest of my life. This traumatised patients, including me. The staff directed us to our rooms and we were medicated. I never learned if the patient survived, but I assumed from the staff reactions that she passed away.

I also experienced the seclusion room. I was in the dining room but did not want to eat a meal, a fairly typical situation when I was depressed. As I left the dining room, a male supervising nurse shoved me backwards and told me to return to my seat. I felt offended by his shove and so I shoved him back. In an instant, I found myself face down on the floor, pinned to the ground with his foot on my head. I was then aware of being in a seclusion room. I felt like a caged animal. At no point did any staff attempt to reason with me or find out what had triggered my reactive outburst. A short while later I yelled to be let out because I had done nothing wrong, I wanted someone to listen to my account of what had occurred. I faced a wall of people who pounced on me and again pinned me to the ground. No one would tell me what was being administered to me, even though I demanded to know. No efforts were made by staff to assist me with my distress. I was given a 'cocktail' of tranquilisers, which knocked me unconscious for several hours.

Even if restraint was required, I refuse to believe that the kinds of bruises I received were necessary. There are holding methods used in many establishments these days that don't leave the patient with such injuries.

In the end, I was worse when I came out of that clinic than when I went in – and I was suicidal when I went in! I experienced profound pain, humiliation, terror, physical harm and hurt during my stay at this particular public hospital, and I certainly did not need any more of this, given my history.

I maintained my job with Kids in Care for seven years. I continued to work, study and complete assignments and field placements. I worked around the clock and twice I collapsed from exhaustion and found myself in hospital for time out. During this time, my biological father committed suicide, and both my biological mother and one of my biological brothers died from cancer.

Five more years passed and, after eight straight years of study, while supporting myself, I received my undergraduate university degree. This was the day that I absolutely, inarguably, gloriously, triumphantly, permanently, successfully and conclusively proved my mother w-r-o-n-g! Good for nothing? I think not. I felt magnificent!

I became the first person in the state of New South Wales to set a precedent outside the Statute of Limitations by some thirty years, and be awarded victims' compensation for abuse sustained as a child while under the care of the State. It was a long road for me, one I never thought I would attempt. My concern and awe in the face of the legal system, my fears of not being believed by the authorities and of my brother-in-law's ability to harm me, had all combined to frighten me away from taking this important step earlier. With the compensation I received, I paid my university fees and all outstanding debts, bought myself a new car and my very own home.

When my work with Marie-Pierre ended, I was living independently and managing my own affairs. My life had taken a giant step forward, and I had begun to believe I really could make my dreams come true. Life beyond abuse, beyond mental illness, became a possibility. All in all, I spent fifteen years working with Marie-Pierre and I cannot adequately express my debt of gratitude for what she helped me achieve over that time.

Although I was still on medication for bipolar disorder, I had been stable for some time. I was holding down a full-time job as a youth worker. I had my degree behind me and I was happy. I thought I was living in someone else's dream.

At work, I chose to transfer to the role of Residential Support Worker, caring for young adults with intellectual disabilities. A year into my new position, my immediate Team Leader became aware of my mental illness. From that moment onward, she went out of her way to make sure I was denied any opportunity to act in a senior capacity or be promoted in any way. Another staff member, who had been informed of my illness, told me I should not be working with the young adults in my care as I was 'ratty, batty and dangerous'! The worker was directed to apologise by management. He did so, reluctantly, but continued to harass and intimidate me.

The worst incident of workplace harassment I endured followed my return to work after a stint in hospital. I walked into the staff office, and those present deliberately looked the other way and left the room. I followed them into the next room and they repeated the behaviour. I told them that I was not contagious. But regardless of how they behaved, they couldn't hurt me badly enough to make me give up. I had come this far. I had fought and I survived. I was determined and had the will to hang on.

I have experienced appalling discrimination, poor treatment and harassment in my private life, too. My neighbour of eight years often took it upon herself, usually when drunk, to call the police to tell them she feared for her life, living next door to a psychiatric patient. On one occasion, she called out to me loudly in the presence of her young son, 'Hey Bipolar, go kill yourself!' I cried for hours. She regularly called me *Bipolar*, as if it were my name. She eventually moved house, but not before telling other neighbours to stay well away from me and smashing three of my four bedroom windows. Thankfully, the kindness of many warm-hearted neighbours outweighs the antagonism I continue to receive from some ignorant individuals. I feel angry and insulted when I hear people refer to the mentally ill as *nutcases*, *lunatics*, *psychos*, *crazies*, *nutters*, or *schizos*. I also believe it is irresponsible behaviour when the media portray the mentally ill as knife-wielding maniacs. These ill-informed journalists only enhance my commitment to conquer prejudice and discrimination and to teach and inform others of mental health issues.

Over twenty years, the side-effects of medication have had a devastating effect on me. I have gained an incredible amount of weight, resulting in medication-induced diabetes. This, in turn, has resulted in other problems. In 2000 I was re-admitted to hospital for severe depression. While there, I was assaulted by an inpatient in the ward, and sustained a blow-out fracture to the right eye. This patient was a martial arts expert, and I required three hours of reconstructive surgery to my face.

I felt defeated, fearful and profoundly depressed, so I reconnected with Marie-Pierre and our work together this time focused on the assault and its immediate effects, with the end goal being a full return to work.

Despite my best efforts, I was unable to cope. I was referred to an independent Government Medical Officer and in 2001 I was medically retired and deemed unfit to work. My career was terminated and my self-esteem diminished. I felt devoid of hope and despondent about my future.

I decided not to let this break my spirit. My case worker suggested I join a social club for people living with a mental illness, that was about to be launched in my community. I became the first member to register with the club. I met some wonderful people, and for the first time in my life I started having fun. In 2006, I tapped into my creative talent and learned how to do quilting. I derived a great sense of satisfaction from making and completing my first quilt, which has since won first and second prize in two separate exhibitions.

I delight in keeping myself busy and maintaining an active mind. I enjoy writing, having coffee at the local café, watching movies, spending time with friends and shopping. I have also redirected my painting skills onto canvas rather than the house! I get a great sense of fulfilment doing this. I spend time with the social network of friends I have built. I can honestly say that those whom I have allowed into my life, and my 'surrogate' family, who mean the world to me, have accepted me for who I am and offer great support.

I have met people recently who find it hard to believe I have a mental illness. Bipolar disorder cannot be seen physically, but I am not ashamed or afraid of having it. It has been a battle, but I manage it. Despite relapses, I have learned better ways to deal with my episodes of pain – by reaching out to those who care for me.

I persevere with taking my medication, but I cannot take antidepressants when I am in my darkest place, as they send me into an instant high. In an elevated state, anything is possible. I have given away substantial amounts of money and personal belongings, run up a credit card, tried to sell my car, had my house valued, mown the lawn at 3 a.m. (!) and engaged in many forms of risk-taking behaviour. When I am down in the zone of depression, I can only 'ride out the wave'.

With the encouragement of my psychiatrist and the local mental health team, I started a local support group for those with mental illness, where I raised funds and donations from local businesses to support group activities. My dream of developing a dedicated website has also been achieved.

I believe in being in charge of my own life: I am the master of my destiny. I accept, trust and believe that our life encounters and events are not our master. We always have a choice. We live in a hurt and damaged world. We simply can't allow setbacks, disappointments, hurt, anger and vengeance to rule our lives or make us bitter. If only we can turn the situation around, we can make something positive of it and learn from the experience. My life has been easier than some people's and harder than others'. I harbour no bitterness, and believe my life experiences were placed in my path for a reason. I don't believe in accidents. Without my personal experiences and mental illness, I doubt I would be the sensitive, caring, generous and compassionate person that I am today.

I don't need the latest modern appliances, a rich bank account, a sports car, a fancy watch or a yacht. I have a life of my own, loving friends, a wonderful surrogate family who genuinely love me, and a therapist who taught me to believe in myself. I have amounted to a very competent and successful individual with self-respect, respect for others, a generous disposition, inner peace and a purpose in life.

Being human can sometimes necessitate being courageous. Nothing can stand in your way if you don't let it.

* * *

Maree is currently writing her own book, *In Someone Else's Dream*.

> I first met Maree in 1985, and was her therapist for over fifteen years.
>
> As you read this magnificent story, you may be tempted to think, 'This couldn't possibly have happened!' Well, it did. This is an inspiring account of one woman's fight to survive, to overcome a past littered with pain and abuse, to build a life for herself, and make a place for herself in society, despite the odds.
>
> Most of all, it is a true account of one woman's immense capacity to love – no matter what. And not let anything stand in the way of a satisfying and fulfilling life.
>
> Marie-Pierre Cleret, Psychotherapist

Two: Tonya

It wasn't until I was well established in my legal career that I first suffered symptoms of bipolar disorder, and I had no idea what was going on.

I was born in Charlotte, North Carolina, into a large family with seven brothers and sisters. My father died when I was very young but other than this I had a great childhood. I had plenty of friends and spent a lot of time playing basketball.

At eighteen, I left home to attend the University of North Carolina for four years and then went on to Ithaca, New York and Cornell Law School. I chose law after working in a law office at the age of fourteen. My mother was a paralegal, a lawyer's assistant, and I was allowed to work in her office. I made copies and typed up documents. I enjoyed working there so much that I decided I wanted to be a lawyer. The idea of taking on cases that helped people appealed to me.

After graduating, I passed the bar and moved to Washington, DC. I first took a position with the Federal Trade Commission doing antitrust law, then joined the Department of Justice as a litigator. It was fabulous work. When the savings and loans industry went belly-up in the eighties, the United States government stepped in and propped them up with various accounting gimmicks. Later on, the government decided not to allow the savings and loans companies to use the accounting gimmicks anymore. When the government repealed the legislation that allowed the use of those gimmicks, many savings and loans organisations sued the United States government, alleging that the government had reneged on its promises.

I was one of many lawyers working on these cases. They were high-profile, high-dollar-value, high-publicity cases. One of my cases was worth eight million dollars, and I worked on another that was worth well over one hundred million dollars. People were very interested in the outcomes.

I worked around the clock. My days were spent in court, cross-examining or examining witnesses, or at depositions. I did a lot of travelling when deposing witnesses and getting ready for trial, because I was also the case handler before things headed to court. I had the opportunity to work on some very high profile cases and I gained a lot of excellent experience. My career was going well.

When I first moved to Washington I was living alone, and although I did go out socially, it wasn't often as I worked such long hours. However, after living in DC for about a year I did meet someone, and we dated for some time before moving in together. We developed what I consider a quiet, stable home life. I was happy. I enjoyed both my home life and the very rewarding work that I was doing. At the time, however, I was under a tremendous amount of stress. It was a very, very stressful job. The hours were long and there was continual pressure to perform at a very high level.

This went on for several years until, when I was about 26 years old, I developed a myriad of symptoms that no one could attribute to any medical cause. I started to experience severe headaches and numbness in my extremities, and I lost a lot of weight. I began to experience paranoia, to believe that people at work were out to get me. One day I curled up on the floor at home, crying uncontrollably, unable to go into the office. Sometimes I would simply not go into the office, for no apparent reason. On other days I would leave at around two o'clock, without telling anybody and without taking leave. I started to behave in an irrational, strange manner and had no idea why. It was scary.

Nobody at work noticed what was going on. It wasn't until the very end of my time there that people recognised that something was wrong. That had a lot to do with the way our office was set up. Litigators worked very independently. We were given our work and trusted to get it done. There was nobody there to babysit us. Our written work was reviewed and we conducted mock hearings before a court attendance, but aside from that there was a vast amount of independence. So it was very easy for people to remain blissfully unaware of other people's concerns.

I struggled with my symptoms for months and months. Being a high achiever, just like my colleagues, my deteriorating health was very hard for me to face. It was devastating. It was just so difficult for me to say, 'Hey, I can't do this anymore,' so I continued to press on believing that I would be fine. I also didn't realise just how ill I was, and didn't want to feel like a failure. So I just kept pushing ahead. Not surprisingly, without any treatment, things at work fell apart and so did my relationship.

My relationship collapsed for a variety of reasons. It came apart because I was ill, and my partner didn't really understand and neither did I. It fell apart because I was working so many hours. It fell apart because I was the primary breadwinner and my partner was accustomed to a certain standard of living that I was providing. If my job was in jeopardy, so was that lifestyle. I ended up very much on my own. It was really difficult.

Eventually, I had to leave the job at the Department of Justice. My health got so bad that I simply had no choice. In the end, I formally resigned twice. The first time I rescinded it. The second time I let it stand and went home.

It's a harsh profession, a hard environment, and this was a very unforgiving group. These very highly motivated, very high achievers were not the most understanding people in the world. There was a lot of work to be done and losing somebody who had my experience meant that they were going to have to try and replace me with somebody who needed to be brought up to speed. They weren't happy about that. I wasn't happy myself, but I had no choice.

So, after seven and a half years, I left and I went home to Charlotte to live with my mother. She was very supportive, but my siblings raised their eyebrows and people we knew certainly wondered what had happened. I didn't provide any answers and neither did my mother.

My mother was the type of person who didn't talk about problems and swept things under the rug. She was the only one I was in contact with prior to coming back, and she was the only person who had any inkling of what was going on with me. Even she had no idea of the extent of what was going on, and neither did I.

After I returned home my symptoms subsided for a while, but they soon returned. At first I wasn't working, so I would only leave the house during the day to do grocery shopping and go to the laundromat. At the laundromat, I began to sense that private messages were being sent to me through the television. When I was at home, I was certain my co-workers were judging me because I had ended up leaving the Department of Justice.

I'm not really sure how, but my sister who works in the mental health field recognised that something wasn't right. During a week when my mother was out of town, my sister asked me to meet her in a public place, our local park. When I arrived, she walked right up to me and said, 'You know, Tonya, it's a beautiful mind. Something is wrong and you need to get help.'

She took me to the hospital that day and told the staff that I was both homicidal and suicidal. I was stunned by this because I didn't want to kill anyone – myself or others – but I didn't challenge what she said because I was afraid and I knew that something was wrong. I was admitted.

That hospital stay was a very frightening event for me. For the first day and a half I just slept. Then I began to get up and venture out of my room. It didn't take me long to realise what it took to get out. You had to go to group sessions and you needed to participate. I had to make people believe that I was making some progress so I could leave. So I 'made progress.' I began to interact with the other patients. I remember one patient in particular who would walk around the unit for exercise; I began to walk with him. We didn't actually talk to each other at all, but we would meet up and do our daily walk together up and down the hallway. There was another patient who had come in after attempting to kill himself by cutting both of his wrists. I remember talking to him about his experience. He was so disappointed in himself for attempting suicide because he had a family and felt that he should never have tried to do something like that. I understood. I was interacting which meant I was getting closer to going home. Soon after, I was on my way out the door.

Things were OK for a while because I was taking medication; however, I hadn't been given a diagnosis. No one ever sat down with me and told me that I had any condition in particular. I do remember seeing something on a piece of paper in my file about depression, so when they released me after eight or nine days, I assumed I was suffering from a bad case of depression and I simply continued with the medication, which seemed to help.

Life continued, relatively symptom-free. I took a teaching job and met a new partner. I took my medication for a while but then stopped as I had difficulty dealing with the side-effects. The medication made me unable to respond sexually and I was very frustrated by that. My relationship was in jeopardy because of it so my solution at the time – a poor one in hindsight – was to stop taking the medication. It didn't affect me right away. I had enough medicine built up in my system that I was OK for a while. But eventually my behaviour became irrational again. I started hearing voices and I became very erratic at work.

My mother was diagnosed with stomach cancer in May 2003 and died in October that same year. It was crushing for me and I went into an episode after her death. My living arrangements changed. I got my own apartment, started living alone and soon found myself back in hospital.

Again I was not given a diagnosis. Staff made sure I took the medication and attended group, but nobody sat down with me to talk about my condition, how to manage it and what was required to get better. Nobody there was practising good medicine. I understand that now, but I didn't realise it back then.

I came away from this hospitalisation understanding that I needed to keep taking medication. It is a life-long thing in my case. I committed myself to staying on the medication, and for the next two years I did very well. For a while I continued teaching and eventually I returned to the practice of law.

And I began to develop symptoms again. I'm not sure what triggered it. I can't identify any one thing. Work was stressful but not excessively so. I was working long hours, but I didn't feel that the hours were too much. I became unable to work and ended up on disability leave. After a while my employer was unable to hold my position and I lost my job.

I was becoming more and more irrational and eventually stopped taking my medication. Then things really started spiralling out of control. I stopped sleeping. For days on end I stayed up all night, writing poetry and working on a book about my life. Then I would crash and burn, sleeping the days away. I experienced delusions and believed I was a producer for the Oprah Winfrey show. I went around telling people that I was one of Oprah's producers. I went to nightclubs to recruit talent for Oprah Winfrey and a new business that she was starting. At one point, I found myself standing at the microphone in a club claiming that I worked for Oprah Winfrey. That night, a friend who knew me was at the nightclub. She saw and heard me at the microphone but she didn't say anything to me about it. Instead, she went home and called another friend and told her what happened. Unfortunately, neither one of them could muster the courage to confront me about my irrationality. No one told me that I was having delusions, so I continued to have them. And they continued to be about Oprah Winfrey.

I went on like this for months. I went on spending sprees. The spending sprees became so outrageous that I stopped paying my mortgage, my car loan and all of my household bills. I took all the money from my retirement account and spent it. I ran up an enormous amount of debt, opening ten new credit card accounts in the space of two months, none of which were being paid. Slowly, my life was unravelling. My mortgage was two, three, then four months late. My car was repossessed and I had to scramble to get it back. My telephones were turned off and my other utilities were in jeopardy of being turned off.

As my life spiralled further and further out of control, my family became more and more alarmed, but not proactive enough to intervene. Eventually I ended up back at the hospital, buzzing like a bee.

I went from person to person seeking attention and demanding their time. Finally, after several days I met a new psychiatrist. He actually sat me down and gave me the diagnosis of bipolar disorder and explained why he thought the diagnosis was accurate. He gave me a prescription for medication and asked me to stay in touch with him.

The medication helped to stabilise me and let me think rationally; and the diagnosis enabled me to finally gather some knowledge about my illness. I conducted a lot of research into the symptoms and treatments, and over time became very knowledgeable about bipolar disorder. This was helpful. Being able to understand my illness and take action really empowered me.

I became very keen to get involved in mental health care and activities and joined the Board of Directors of National Alliance on Mental Illness (NAMI) in North Carolina to make sure that the rights of people with mental illness were protected. I also sit on the NAMI Education Committee. In that capacity I'm responsible for educating consumers and the public about mental illness.

There's an incredible stigma created around mental illness and it makes it very difficult to work, difficult to date and difficult to live. I am a mature, intelligent, educated, professional woman, but facing the challenge of mental illness is hard in a society where people just don't understand. Despite this I'm doing well. Although I occasionally have relapses, I've been very well for over a year now.

Finding an outlet for having fun in my life is an aspect I'm still struggling with. During the time when my life spiralled out of control, a lot of friends distanced themselves and decided to have nothing more to do with me. I'm still adjusting to that in some cases, though there were a few who stayed in my life.

I don't have a partner at the moment. That's tough and I've been trying to figure out how to move forward in this part of my life. I am a lesbian woman and that's alienating enough in a small community. But when you add mental illness, and the need to disclose that to people who are close to me, the universe becomes even smaller. I still hold out hope. I view dating again as part of my total recovery.

The road to recovery has been really difficult for me because of the enormous losses I've had to endure. For a long time I was very depressed and seriously contemplating ending it all. I got to the point of doing research on the internet to establish whether the medication I was taking would kill me if I took enough of it. I didn't really want to die. It was just that the circumstances were so terrible and hard to face. But by doing that research, I started finding other things to read. I found accounts that were uplifting and encouraging from other people with mental illness. This gave me something precious beyond price – hope.

Once I had a sense of hope I realised that I could come back from this, with knowledge. And knowledge is power. This is what spurred me to read everything I could lay my hands on and understand as much as I could about the illness.

So my recovery started with a spark of hope. Feeling hope gave me empowerment, and it was this empowerment and self-education that put me on the road to recovery.

I became involved with a support group and through this, with helping other people. Being out there and educating the public about mental illness and participating in the various NAMI initiatives gave me a sense of purpose.

I am working again now, and I write a monthly column about health issues for an internet magazine. This month I wrote a piece called 'My Son's Keeper', about a woman whose son has schizophrenia. I've also written my own story, an article called 'Coming Out of the Shadows: Living with Bipolar Disorder'.

To anyone out there facing mental health issues, I encourage you to educate yourself. Being educated is so very important. You need to know all you can about your illness, medication and treatment options.

Secondly, I suggest you find a good psychiatrist. I have a really wonderful psychiatrist and I cannot emphasise the benefits of this enough. The relationship between the individual and the psychiatrist is very important to recovery and healing.

Finally, I encourage you to find hope. Read everything you can about people who have overcome similar challenges to the ones you face. Read, talk and listen and find that spark of hope that you need to start taking control of your life again.

Three: Julie

I believe I was born with bipolar disorder.

Even as a child I was always angry and frustrated. I was terribly shy and self-conscious, extremely so, and always felt 'different'. Always at a loss to understand why I didn't feel happy like other people, I believed I was simply a terrible person and not as worthy as others.

My parents were constantly fighting when I was young. There was never peace in our home. My father would fly into terrible rages and hit my mother, knocking her to the floor and hurting her. I was the eldest of four children and, as I grew older, he would take his temper out on me also.

In my teens, in addition to anger, frustration and shyness, I started to experience depression. My family history is riddled with bipolar disorder and mental illnesses, but back then I wasn't aware of it.

At the age of eighteen, I was diagnosed with manic depression (now known as bipolar disorder). The language used in 1966 differed greatly from today: I was told that I was a 'manic depressive'. I understood that I would need tablets all my life. My doctors did everything they could to help me, but so much less was known about bipolar disorder back then.

During my first hospitalisation, I was given three courses of electro-convulsive therapy, known commonly as 'shock treatment,' but it was unsuccessful for me. The use of electro-convulsive therapy has changed over the years, and I understand that it is now a much safer and more effective procedure, but it was not appropriate for my condition.

The depression I experienced was so deep and so dark that I would scream out in anguish and pain. I could barely stand it. The mental torment was more agonising to me than any physical injury could ever be. I lost the will to live and attempted suicide more times than I can count.

Then the mania would come and take me so high that reality would become a blur, and eventually disappear. Mania is wonderful to feel but, in truth, is even more dangerous and damaging than depression.

A complete breakdown would follow. I've had several. I've been institutionalised more times than I care to remember. And that's what my experience with bipolar is. Huge swings between extreme, overwhelming highs and devastating lows. It's agony.

There is no line in the sand between mentally ill and mentally well, with everyone belonging on either one side or the other. I see our mental and emotional functioning as a continuum, a line like a piece of string. Those who operate within the mid-section of the line are the 'functional majority' and those who operate a little further out, at either end at any given time, are less functional. Much of my life has been spent at the extreme ends, swinging back and forth.

When I was young, my mother warned me never to tell anyone what was wrong with me, as mental illness has a stigma and others would think I was 'queer'. So I became adept at covering up. After stints in hospital, friends would ask what was wrong with me, so I would say 'I'm not sure, they can't quite put their finger on it,' and the questions would stop. Of course, people still knew I was different.

Many people simply have not believed that I am mentally ill – surely I was merely moody and lacking self-control. Those who did believe I had a mental illness thought of me as 'crazy' and avoided me at all costs. Many well-intentioned people believed that I could be completely healed simply by following their advice and applying willpower. It's *mind over matter,* apparently.

Needless to say, they were extremely disappointed with me when

I failed. These were some of the darkest periods of my life. Of course, my family and friends did not and could not understand the nature of what I was going through, despite their belief to the contrary. They were always well-intentioned and I am grateful that they loved me enough to try. I appreciate how devastating a mental illness can be for family, friends and loved ones.

To overcome my extreme shyness, my mother suggested I write to the Lonely Hearts' Club. I was only twenty years old at the time, so I sent in a photo and was inundated with letters! Many of them I didn't answer, but one stood out from the pack: Alan from Brisbane. He was 6 feet 5 inches tall – a giant of a man – and he seemed so nice. We wrote at first, and then started talking on the phone. We stayed in touch by phone, even during my hospitalisations.

I eventually travelled to Brisbane to meet him, and we fell in love. He was actually a notorious criminal, but at the time I had no idea. He ran prostitution rings and smuggled stolen goods, but I didn't know that until well after we were married. I also hadn't realised that Alan was an angry and violent man. The physical and emotional abuse began early.

When I fell pregnant, Alan was furious. He held me down and attacked me ferociously in an attempt to abort the baby. It was a terrifying and agonising experience, but the pregnancy continued and I delivered a healthy baby girl.

To his surprise, Alan found that he quite liked our daughter, Sonya, when she was born, but he quickly became extremely jealous of her, so the situation remained tenuous. I left him once, when the baby was about fifteen months old, but then foolishly went back to see if things could be worked out. I made the same mistake that so many women make. I believed his apology would matter for more than a day. I believed that he would work hard and maybe actually change.

Things went well at first but then, after only a few weeks, the beatings started again with vigour! Alan didn't want me to spend any time with the baby. He had no patience with her and would bellow, 'Shut that kid up!' whenever she cried. Our daughter was terrified of him. If she was alone with him in a room, she would fall silent, curl up on the floor and bury her face. By this time, Alan was beating me several times a week and my self-esteem was almost completely destroyed.

Until the night that he took Sonya away from me. He wanted me to focus on being a good wife to him, without the baby's interference. Having my child taken from me was the one thing I simply couldn't stand. But he enjoyed every minute of it. He would grin and taunt me. 'Not so happy now, are ya?'

I was devastated. I developed a terrible migraine and could barely cope, but I was determined to take my baby and escape! I acted as happy and carefree as I was able for the next two days. I showed no signs of being unhappy or acting out of the ordinary in any way.

I was fairly certain that he had taken the baby to his sister's house, so I put a plan in motion. I called my father and elder brother, who agreed to drive all night to reach Brisbane, take me to my sister-in-law's house once Alan had left for work the next day, grab the baby and leave Brisbane immediately.

As planned, my father arrived the next morning after Alan left for work, and I quickly gathered the most important of my things. We drove to my sister-in-law's house and, sure enough, there was Sonya, eating an ice-cream with my two little nieces. As soon as she saw me arrive, my sister-in-law phoned Alan to alert him. I grabbed the baby and got out of the house. I never saw Alan again.

My mother was pleased to have me back home. I divorced Alan on the grounds of mental cruelty and physical abuse. Many people believed that his abuse had been my fault. Because of 'the way I was', surely I must have driven the poor man to it. I was a hysterical woman and I clearly deserved it. Violence against women wasn't considered important back then.

Once I arrived back home, I had a complete nervous breakdown. It was my first but certainly not my last. I didn't see a doctor about this one. I just survived it somehow and I balanced out again over time.

Unfortunately, the situation in the family home was almost as bad. Following her divorce from my father, my mother had married Lewin, my stepfather. Lewin was aggressive and extremely abusive. Once I was in the house, he tried to pressure me into having sex with him – of course I refused. He was impossible to live with and was cruel to my mother. He had an affair with my brother's wife, which enraged and devastated my brother and tore our family apart for years to come.

My brother's wife had been sexually abused by her uncle since she was a child and I believe that she was just as damaged as the rest of us.

My mother had to 'tiptoe on eggshells', given the bad blood in the family. The tension of those times is simply indescribable. My mother left my stepfather, took those of us still living with her (my two youngest siblings were still teenagers) and moved to a housing commission flat on the outskirts of town.

As we lived in a small town, it didn't take long for my stepfather to find us. He came over one afternoon and was talking with my mother when my brother arrived for a visit. He recognised our stepfather's car and, remaining outside, shouted for him to come outside and face him. My brother was barely in control, and it was clear that if the two met, there would be bloodshed, if not murder.

My mother was so distressed she told my stepfather to leave immediately, and she threw his keys outside into the dirt. She then started pleading with my brother. 'Don't hit him, it's not worth it. He'll have you arrested and where will that leave us? Please, please don't hit him,' she begged.

'You have five minutes to get out of this house alive!' my brother shouted through the door. Eventually, after a highly tension-filled exchange, my mother standing between them, my stepfather got into his car and left. We all found the tension of this situation absolutely unbearable. And events of this nature kept happening again and again.

Life was very hard. I was sexually promiscuous and drifted from one relationship to the next. I began to abuse alcohol regularly and developed a serious drinking problem that lasted for some years. I was 'quietly' drunk almost every day and would drink to unconsciousness on weekends.

My drinking really only subsided when my stepfather died suddenly of heart failure and we moved from the country town to a major city. I was then away from my previous boyfriend and the 'good time' social circle that supplied my alcohol. A pensioner, I could no longer afford to purchase alcohol myself. But I craved it, strongly, for several more years.

I have been heavily medicated, institutionalised and locked in padded cells. I've been desperate to die many times, simply to end the pain. It was so severe at times that I believed I'd be driven mad by it. I cannot accurately describe the total and unrelenting effort it has been simply to get by day by day, hour by hour and minute by minute. I was prescribed up to seventy-five tablets a day to keep me stable, and have tried too many different medications over the years to count. The side-effects that accompanied those early drugs were something to behold. To this day there are long periods of my life of which I have no recollection. There are years that have been completely lost but, by the grace of God, I got by.

In 1980 at the age of thirty-two, I experienced my first visual hallucination. I was terrified. Strangely enough, though I had never hallucinated before, I knew it was about to happen. I could actually feel that it was about to start. It came with a loud clanging noise and the images I saw – worthy of an Academy Award as a bloodcurdling horror movie – remain clear in my memory to this day.

My mother believed it was a dream. Unfortunately, it wasn't. I had been awake. I experienced a spate of these visual hallucinations for some months. I saw children playing, just like a moving portrait on what was in fact a blank wall, and various other images.

Thankfully, with medication and effective avoidance strategies, I have rarely experienced visual hallucinations since. I did, however, start hearing and smelling things that weren't there, and I still do. I sometimes hear noises, such as a wooden door falling on the ground, but most often I hear people's voices. Some are known to me and others aren't. Sometimes I can hear a garbled, unintelligible message, but other times I hear clear words and phrases. I once heard my brother tell me he was going to 'turn the key and open the wall'. Often the voices are simply calling my name.

I have heard distorted voices coming from cats. Many of these I recognise as hallucinations, although sometimes a human voice I know can fool me. But this holds no fear at all for me now.

I developed schizoaffective disorder (features of both bipolar disorder and schizophrenia) in 1980, and it was diagnosed in 1982. I was often out of control and violent, sometimes towards people but more often towards material things, such as public phone boxes. I was not thinking rationally and was unable to control my rage. I have always believed that depression is anger turned inwards on yourself. I know this to be true, as I have actually felt this transformation of outward anger turning to inward depression.

It was around this time that my ex-husband, Alan, hired a private detective to find me. He was thirty-eight years old and dying of bone cancer. My daughter was thirteen, and neither of us had seen or heard from him since we fled those years before. Regardless of our history, I was shocked at the news that Alan was dying at such a young age. I was devastated and cried for days.

Alan asked me to come and see him before he died, but I refused. Then he asked to see Sonya. Knowing how dangerous Alan was, I desperately didn't want her to go. But he was sick and she wanted to meet her father, so she travelled to Brisbane in the care of my mother and eldest brother. Alan died two years later.

I met my second husband at a psychiatric hospital. We were both inpatients and well out of touch with reality at the time. His delusions were much more powerful than any I had experienced. For a time he believed himself to be the reincarnation of King David. Given the circumstances, it is not surprising that the marriage did not last long. Matters were not helped by his insistence that we live with his mother throughout the marriage. His mother did not approve of me, so this caused a lot of problems. My husband and I continued a physical relationship for many years following our divorce and, although this has now ceased, we remain firm friends to this day.

It was a tumultuous relationship but there was only one instance of physical violence, which occurred when he was extremely ill and out of control. He struck me in the face and head – only twice, but the blows were so exceptionally hard that I barely retained consciousness. Since this time, he has recovered completely and has experienced no symptoms of mental illness for over twenty years. His mother has now passed on and he is in a healthy relationship with a lovely woman. I wish them well.

With age and experience, I became increasingly adept at managing my illness. I made the conscious choice to live alone so I could manage my own needs in a way that was not disruptive or destructive to others. My daughter remained living with my mother, to provide stability; and I continued to see my daughter daily.

I still suffered greatly. In 1997 I intended to kill myself through electrocution but, for a number of reasons, I didn't go ahead. It was around this time that I began to really develop my faith in God.

My third marriage was to a man many years older than me, who developed both dementia and mental illness late in life. I clearly remember the morning that he dressed himself to leave the house in nothing but a pair of ladies' pantyhose, a woollen jumper and gumboots. I considered stopping him, but realised that it was only by being picked up by the police that he would be forced to get help. So I let him go without comment. I really shouldn't laugh but honestly, it looked absolutely hilarious. Obscene but hilarious. I can find humour in most things, which is a strategy that has held me in good stead over the years. Of course, he was picked up by the police shortly afterwards and admitted to hospital for a period of time.

He died of stroke about twelve months later. His loss devastated me, as have each of the losses I experienced throughout my life. I have never been able to manage grief effectively, and this remains my greatest struggle to this day.

I then found Colin, the love of my life. This relationship was special from the outset. Everyone was delighted for me when I met him – he was so charming that everyone liked him. It was something that just felt *right* for both of us, and we fell in love quickly. He moved in with me and we spent most of our time together. He was a genuinely kind and loving person. He devoted himself to helping everyone around him: nothing was too much trouble. He suffered from schizophrenia and we found that we really understood each other. We were able to share our deepest thoughts and feelings. We were soul mates.

But only weeks into the relationship, in the middle of the night, he got out of bed, struggling for breath. He fell and died right there on our bedroom floor.

The next day, his grown children came to the house and took all of his belongings. I wanted to keep in touch but they said that they didn't want to see or hear from me again.

Of the hundreds of people I have met in institutions over the years, none are quite as sad perhaps as young people who have become mentally ill through recreational drug use. It amazes me that people are willing to risk permanently changing their brain chemistry and becoming mentally ill.

My last suicide attempt in 2005 was the closest I came to success.

I took over five hundred tablets and was unconscious for three days. Though it sounds like a lot, with the number of pills I was taking at the time, amassing five hundred of them was hardly a challenge. I was beside myself with pain at the time. I believe that I am at my most selfish when suicidal. I am unwilling and unable to consider anyone other than myself at these times, and this is something I have often deeply regretted. Thankfully, I have moved past a lot of my selfishness these days.

Grief remains my greatest trial. Grief and loss. I suffer to this day with what is termed 'bad grief' – long-term, unresolved and highly painful. I have lost so many people who were dear to me that when my grief 'comes on', I find the pain excruciating. The greatest loss of all to bear was my mother's death. When I feel down these days, it is often due to grief, in addition to my illness.

I have a number of distinct mental illnesses. I have had bipolar disorder from a very young age and developed schizoaffective disorder at the age of thirty-two. Then in my fifties, I was diagnosed with borderline personality disorder and chronic generalised anxiety disorder.

I am sixty-one years old now, and physically I am not in the best shape. I suffer from asthma, poor eyesight, irritable bowel syndrome, chronic fatigue syndrome and high blood pressure. I also suffer from advanced rheumatoid and osteoarthritis in my spine, hands and feet, and require daily doses of morphine to manage the pain.

Despite these challenges, I can tell you with honesty that I have found great peace and joy in my life at last. I accept my illnesses, and from this has come great healing. I now attempt to approach life with an 'ease' and 'flow' rather than a fight and struggle. I know that I am not my illnesses and that, although I may never be free of all mental illness, I lead a rich and happy life most of the time.

Recently a memory came back to me, from fifty years ago. I remembered my mother yelling at my father, calling him names and telling him he had a 'yellow streak'. As a child I had no idea what that meant, but I knew it was something bad. He struck my mother hard and knocked her to the ground. I believe this was a critical moment for me, perhaps even the very moment that I took on the oppressive stress that I have struggled with ever since. With the return of this memory came the realisation that I don't have to carry that stress any more.

I have also remembered an early moment of complete exasperation. I felt enraged. I remember becoming aware that anger was not socially acceptable, and in that instant the anger left. It was soon replaced by depression. Now I realise that I have no need to repress my feelings any more.

I wear rings that commemorate all of the important relationships I have been blessed with throughout my life. The most beautiful ring of all commemorates my relationship with Colin. I never ask God why he was taken. Instead I thank God so very much for giving us that beautiful time together. I have a deep personal connection with God, and this brings me great comfort. His love and grace are beyond comparison.

I have developed profound insight and understanding from my life's experiences. I hold no grudges against others and I forgive fully and completely. I am able to do this because I have recognised a simple truth: we are all doing our best. With limits, faults, flaws and less-than-perfect understanding, certainly; but this doesn't matter. By and large, we are all doing our best with what we know and have available to us.

This is why arguments are completely pointless. You may tell someone that they have done things wrong and you are extremely angry. It is human nature for them to feel as though they did their best and fail to see what they might have done differently. They will feel hurt and defensive. Who gains from this?

To truly appreciate that everyone has their struggles but we're all basically good people doing our utmost – and extending the same kindness and understanding to ourselves – helps release us from resentment and judgement. I feel love and compassion for others and have a deep sense that we are all connected. In fact, I know we are.

I am not currently in a romantic relationship, and feel at peace with my decision to enjoy my life just as it currently is. Given my previous promiscuous behaviour, I found this change a struggle at first.

I attend grief counselling and also find meditation extremely helpful. Through meditation, I am able to 'quieten the mind' and achieve an inner peacefulness that brings with it a feeling of true joy.

I take much better care of my health these days and ensure I get uninterrupted sleep at night, whenever possible. The benefit of this cannot be overestimated.

In stark opposition to my shy beginnings, I am an absolute extrovert now and am very active. Activity is very healing for me and, regardless of the physical, mental and emotional challenges, I pursue the things in life that bring me fulfilment and joy.

I was, until recently, a proud member of the Harmony of Heart and Minds Community Choir in South Australia and contributed to recording a CD for commercial release. I intend to undertake tertiary study at the local TAFE College.

I have an active, even hectic, social life and I am usually in the company of friends. I realise that going out and mixing with others brings me great happiness. I love watching comedies and listening to classical music. I play the piano and piano accordion (though I don't often find time) – I was a talented artist/painter in my youth. I have close bonds with my family and a particularly close bond with my eldest brother, daughter and grandchildren. I love them intensely and am grateful that none of my children suffer from mental illness.

I don't stop taking my medications when I am well. The fact that I keep taking my medication contributes to my remaining well, though it does not entirely remove my symptoms and it doesn't stop me from relapse. I understand that I need to continue taking medication for life, but I am glad to be living in an age where it is available. The modern medications have far fewer side-effects than the older ones, such as Largactil (I nearly choked to death) and Modocate. I take only a quarter of the amount of medication I used to, and many of my daily pills now are for age-related issues, such as hormone replacement therapy.

I am rather eccentric but I don't care what others think of me. Young people often laugh at me in the street but I don't mind. I am who I am and I accept other people for who they are.

I take the time to thank people for their efforts, even when doing so isn't a typical practice, and I've found this has a profoundly positive impact.

These days I take life in my stride most of the time. If it's anything I have no power over, I accept things and trust God's will. I fear nothing and no one: that's a wonderful feeling.

We are all different, but it is my sincere hope that you will find an approach to healing that is beneficial for you. I am still mentally ill and this means that sometimes I suffer terribly. But most of the time I am well and can honestly say that at last, I am genuinely happy.

Accept. Relax. Believe.

I wish every one of you love, laughter and peace.

God Bless.

Four: Susana

I was eighteen years old when I first developed symptoms of a mood disorder. I began feeling very depressed and stopped enjoying activities I had previously loved. My mother was the only person who saw the difference in my mood, and we initially put it down to my uncertainty about what to study after high school.

Having been born and raised in Argentina, I was thrilled when, at the age of twenty, I won a scholarship to continue my studies in the United States. I was overjoyed, as was my family. This experience started as a great opportunity, but after only four months it came to an abrupt end when I experienced a psychotic episode.

I had not been sleeping well and was eating very little when I commenced studies in the USA. Four months into the course, my class was scheduled to visit an international school in Washington DC. I had not slept at all the previous night and had started feeling very unwell. When I mentioned that to my teacher, she insisted that I have a shower and be ready to attend with the rest of the group.

While in the shower, I thought that I received a message of peace from a higher power and I was given responsibility to deliver this message to the world. I decided to arrange a meeting with the President of the United States of America. I thought it was great luck that the White House was so close. Also beneficial was the fact that press and media representatives would be present that very afternoon!

Upon arrival at the school I told my teachers about my plan for an afternoon meeting with the President and requested that the media cover this world event. The lecturer immediately became concerned about my strange behaviour and took appropriate action. I was very cooperative as two large men escorted me to a paddy wagon and delivered me to the emergency room of the local hospital. On arrival I was sedated to unconsciousness and, to be honest, it was the best sleep I'd had in months. While in hospital I continued to hallucinate, which led to a misdiagnosis of schizophrenia.

In 1980, treatment for mental health was not what it is today. At that time, every illness in the USA that involved psychotic episodes was diagnosed as schizophrenia. As a result, the medication was unsuitable and I remained in a manic condition. I was extremely talkative and socialised extensively with the other patients. I sang, talked and even shared photos with everyone. My mood escalated to the point where I lost touch with reality.

I was eventually released and returned to college. Unfortunately the manic behaviour continued so it was decided that I must be sent back to Argentina. My parents were devastated by the news and my manic mood ended in a deep and long depression.

I became incapable of making decisions for myself due to the serious state of the depression, so my family took me to a psychiatrist. Months of treatment followed, including psychotherapy three times a week, but my condition continued to worsen. I deteriorated to the point that I had to be cared for 24 hours a day.

I spent ten months in bed taking a cocktail of medications that not only didn't help the situation, but contributed to a 25-kilogram weight gain. My negative thinking and low self-esteem drove me to a suicide attempt.

When summer came around, my family decided to holiday at a village near the beach. I did not want to go, and I particularly did not want to be seen in a swimming suit. Each day my mother stayed with me and begged me to go the beach with everyone else. One day she had enough and decided to stop begging. She said, 'You know where we are; when you are ready come and see us.'

Something snapped in my mind. I decided that my mother didn't want me living in this world as I had become a burden. So once she had gone, I closed the door tightly, turned on the gas and went to sleep. I don't know how long I had been dozing when a neighbour saved my life. She was screaming loudly through the door, telling me that gas was leaking. I woke up and eventually turned off the gas.

My family did not know of this incident until many years later; but nonetheless they were worried about my mental state and took me to see another doctor. He was amazed at how many different medications I had been given and believed these were not right for a 21-year-old. He reduced my medication, leaving only the antidepressants.

Reducing my medication slowly brought back enough alertness that I could start a diet and exercise program, known to help lift depression. Gradually the medication became unnecessary.

When I turned 22, my brother Daniel was killed in a car accident. It was deeply shocking – devastating. We were only eleven months apart and he was my only brother. It was so very hard; I was sad every time his name was spoken.

I had plans to get married and come to Australia, but after this tragedy, I had to first revive my mother. Her pain was so great that I thought she would never survive Daniel's death. I took her to a doctor but nothing seemed to help her cope. Eventually, I gave her a shake. I told her that I knew she was struggling but I asked her if she was going to be here for me. That woke her up and she became able to move on.

I managed to regain a normal life with the support of my family and for the next few years my life went on without any major symptoms of a mood disorder. I finished my studies and married Osvaldo, an architect, in 1983. We came to Australia three weeks later on a special visa.

Arriving at Sydney airport was quite a cultural shock. The customs staff were very rude and showed us no respect whatsoever. They took my husband's shoes without explanation and even tried on my clothes without asking permission. They checked every single item in our luggage and explained nothing. I was very tired so I just let them do what they chose without complaint.

We had been told that someone from the Immigration Department would meet us and direct us to our accommodation. But at the end of this long journey, there was no one waiting for us. We didn't know anyone so we just kept waiting for hours. Finally we contacted the police station and a woman came to help us. She called two taxis. I didn't know where they were taking us and I insisted on travelling in my husband's taxi rather than in the second taxi with the luggage. After an hour of driving, we ended up in a hostel. The taxi driver was very nice to us as he was a migrant himself. It was now midnight but he waited with us until we found the manager and were given a key.

Then the next morning at about 7 a.m., a lady with a wheelbarrow came into our apartment and spoke, but I did not understand a word. We were moved to live with a Chilean family, sharing an apartment. I was quite comfortable sharing but the food was terrible and I got ulcers from eating it. It was one thing after another.

The next set-back came when I asked the Commonwealth Employment Service (CES) to assist me in finding a job. When I mentioned that I had a background in Early Childhood, they were completely disinterested and asked what else I could do. I insisted that I could be a school assistant, but they registered me to work as an administrative assistant and bookkeeper.

Things changed for the better after nine weeks of intensive briefing sessions for the newly arrived. We were told how to find a house, how the health system worked and so on. I found these sessions very helpful.

I returned to the CES to express my unhappiness at not being allowed to register for a job in the early childhood field, and to my surprise I discovered that there was a program available for migrant women to work with young children in the multicultural sector. The closing day for applications was that afternoon, so I immediately submitted an application together with my CV. I got an interview and was offered the job. This was my first job at a Community Centre that ran ESL (English as a Second Language) classes; I looked after the children while their parents attended the sessions. My skills were soon recognised and I was offered a better position.

I also received training in multiculturalism, which was advantageous. In the meantime, I applied to the Department of Education to validate my qualifications. After nine months of having to present all sorts of programs, attend interviews and even have x-rays, I was given qualifications equivalent to those of an Australian pre-school or primary teacher. This was a wonderful moment, and I was extremely happy.

I became a teacher's aide before having my first child, Alan, in 1983. Upon my return from maternity leave, I took on a director's role with the responsibility to establish a childcare centre.

Developing a childcare centre with a very small budget, in a tight timeframe with limited help, was an interesting and challenging learning experience but I succeeded. I ran the child care centre for eight years, during which time I had my second child, Veronica, in 1990. It was difficult to raise two children as my husband and I were both employed full-time and had no extended family in Australia.

A year after Veronica's birth, I applied for another job that required the establishment of a new childcare centre, and again, won the position. I went to one of my favourite places on a two-day vacation by myself before I started, to regain the energy needed to tackle the new role ahead of me.

Again, I set up the childcare centre from scratch. This involved planning, budgeting, ordering furniture, developing job descriptions, interviewing staff and so on. I had a deadline of only six weeks. I met the challenge, and the centre opened on time and on budget. I stayed as director for five years and built an excellent team. That is, until December 1996. I was thirty-seven years old and I had no idea at the time that my career as a director was soon to be over.

One morning, I woke up and felt unwell. I thought I had the flu. I had planned to attend a meeting with the council that day, but I was unable to go so I arranged for another teacher to attend in my place. Over the course of that morning, I deteriorated and ended up curled in a foetal position on the stairs of my house. I stayed there for two days.

My husband took me to the doctor, who said that I was extremely depressed and referred me to a clinic. At the time of my admission I was in a catatonic state. I remained in the clinic for nine months.

The nurses were wonderful. They showered and fed me as I was unable to do it myself. I have no memory of this time at all. I don't even remember the transition from consciousness to the foetal position. My brain just shut down.

I was given two medications initially but they didn't work. This was the very worst time of my life. I had to wait ten to fifteen days for each medication to work, and had to be weaned off one before being able to take the other. This time without effective medication was pure hell. I screamed at the nurses, begging them to end my pain. 'I can't bear anymore! I don't want anymore! Please, give me anything. Anything to get me out of this!' I was desperate.

I fully understand how people who are at this stage, outside of a clinic and with no support, attempt suicide. Depression can be extremely painful both mentally and physically, and you can see no way out. It is the raw intensity of this pain that gives people the desire to end their lives. They don't necessarily want to die but they are desperate for the pain to end and feel they have no other choice. That is how it was for me. It was unbearable, absolutely unbearable.

Everything was negative, everything was black. My husband brought a walkman to the clinic and all I could do was lie in bed, listen to the music and sleep. It was a truly horrible time. I believed I was a burden to society. No one needed me and everyone would survive without me. The only thing that kept me alive was a picture of my children that I kept in a frame next to my bed. When I hit rock bottom, I'd pick up the frame and talk to them. I'd say, 'You were not born to be without a mother in this world. I'm going to go through this, no matter how bad the pain gets, to still be with you.'

The doctor suggested we try ECT (electro-convulsive therapy) and my husband was consulted. A second opinion, from a professor of the clinic, confirmed the treatment plan. I had six sessions, one every second day. The treatment began very early in the morning at about five a.m., when I was still half asleep, and it was absolutely OK with me. At that stage, if the doctor had told me that putting my head down a toilet and flushing it would help, I would have done it. I was willing to try anything to find a solution.

ECT was not painful. It was not traumatic. It helped me to get better. ECT was my saviour. One of the side-effects was the loss of short-term memory, but it wasn't extensive and I didn't want to remember the bad things anyway. After the treatments I was taken back to bed to recover from the general anaesthetic and was given breakfast in bed. The first five ECT sessions were fine – they really helped – but the sixth was one too many. By that time I was feeling much better and this final session sent me to the manic side.

The doctor came to me and said, 'Susana, I am now one hundred percent sure of your diagnosis. You have bipolar mood disorder; and that makes you a lucky person because although we cannot cure it, it is a completely manageable condition.'

I thought he must be joking – how could I be a lucky person after all this pain? But he was positive, and assured me that if I followed his treatment plan I'd be fine. This is a moment that I have always remembered because it was the beginning of a positive attitude for me. This was the greatest doctor on earth. He saved my life.

I was extremely happy for about three months. The doctors finally began to realise that being talkative and sociable was not me at all. It was then discovered that one of my manic symptoms was feelings of grandeur.

One day I was in the clinic lounge area, watching television, and saw an advertisement for a glamour photo shoot. I thought this was absolutely fantastic. I immediately booked myself in. I would feel like a queen and I could hardly wait. I convinced another patient to take me in his car and off we went together. He spent three hours waiting for me! Thankfully he was very patient.

I had the time of my life. I had my hair up, down, curled, straightened. The camera just kept flashing everywhere. There was makeup, clothing changes: it was fantastic.

Three weeks later I took three people from the clinic with me to view the photos. There we were, four in a convertible, going to a posh place to view glamour photos. The driver of the car was manic, as was I, so it all seemed great fun. We all agreed on one of the photos and I paid $500 without a moment's hesitation. I had completely lost my understanding of the value of money, that it is an asset to be carefully managed. Even if the photos had cost $1,000, I would have paid it. At this point my husband started to worry, and realised that something was terribly wrong with me. All credit cards soon disappeared from my wallet.

My husband is more action-oriented than a talker. He was as practical as ever and looked after the children. He didn't tell the schoolteachers any details as he wasn't sure how they might react. He didn't want to put the children at risk of a stigma. But he never lied to the children about what was wrong with me. He brought them to the clinic to see me. The children were five and eight years old at the time, and he explained what was happening in a gentle, honest and age-appropriate way. My son and daughter still remember those visits, as they loved playing with the pool table at the clinic. Sometimes when they visited we would go to a local park.

It was a very difficult time for my husband emotionally and financially, as my income had suddenly ceased. Thankfully, we had made mortgage payments one year in advance, so that was very helpful. My husband managed very well for nine months, largely single-handed. My mother-in-law came to help for a month; and my mother came over from Argentina but could only stay for fifteen days. She did not understand my illness at all; she had been in denial since the onset. She didn't ask me about the illness and I believe she may have even felt guilty for having created a child who was suffering as I was.

My behaviour continued to be erratic. I remember a particular night at the clinic. I couldn't sleep and had high levels of energy, so I went to the laundry, moved each machine by myself and scrubbed every spot in the room. Unbelievable! What I didn't notice was that I had left fluff in the sink and the tap was still running. In fact, I flooded the room, the corridor and the entire unit – but the laundry was very clean. Sometimes I would wash my hair at 3 a.m. and then blow-dry it, believing that if I didn't dry it immediately I would catch a cold. I didn't realise that my actions woke up people throughout the entire ward.

But the old rule applied. Everything that goes up must come down, and for the rest of the nine months I was struggling with depression again. It was very deep at times, but I was released from the clinic at this point. I was not fully recovered but I was able to manage and I had a family at home to support me.

When I was sick I thought there was no room in my head to receive any information. I only started to read and gather information when I felt better. At the clinic, I began sourcing as much information as I could. I wanted to learn all I could about how to manage bipolar disorder.

When I was finally discharged, I was told about a support group and decided to try it. I learned a great deal from the members. We shared our feelings and experiences with each other. It was run by a wonderful woman who had a daughter with bipolar disorder. She and her husband had started the group themselves, and she had run it for the previous twenty years. This lady was eighty years old when I first met her.

Over the coming five years, she began losing her hearing. As I was now well, she took me aside and asked me to take over the group as she was unable to continue. So I did. I received help when I was in need, so I feel that it's only right that I, in turn, help others. I've now been running the support group for the last three and a half years. We meet once a month. Attendance numbers fluctuate – sometimes eight people come, sometimes up to 25. I am prepared and always provide tea and coffee for 25 people, and I always take very nice biscuits! I am supported by the Mental Health Association of NSW, and there is a small allowance provided for phone calls (and biscuits!).

I continued with my psychological treatment and undertook cognitive behaviour therapy as an outpatient for ten months after discharge. I attended for four full days each week. Recovery was very difficult and it took me nearly two years to feel OK again. Finally getting there was a great feeling. I was also prescribed the correct medication and the correct dosage. I found that I became a bit slower then I used to be, when taking the medication. I still take the same dosage of medication today but I have no wish to be any faster.

I learned that I have to be patient and care for myself. In the beginning, making dinner at home seemed such a challenge that I made it the most important goal of the day. An achievement! I learned to lie down and have a rest when necessary and listen to the pace of my body and brain. It felt like I had been born again and had to learn everything step by step, from crawling to walking.

I couldn't go back to the work I'd been doing. For fifteen years I had been a director of childcare centres. I was an organised, intelligent, skilled and accomplished woman, and my work was still available to me. However, my doctor suggested I not return, as such stressful work could trigger an episode.

My husband took the time to understand what mental illness is about. He supports me whether I am well or not. When I'm unwell he encourages me; he reminds me that the medication will only do so much and that I need to pull myself through.

When I finally recovered, he opened a conveyancing business and gave me the opportunity to help. I felt that my life was starting again. Like a child, I was scared to get in the car. I became hesitant about a lot of things, but my husband was patient and very helpful. He taught me how to assist with settlements, from an office in the city. He travelled with me on the train, showed me the buildings, pointed out where to get off the train and so on. For someone who had once worked in senior positions and travelled on her own, this was really, truly, starting from scratch. But I got there.

It's been ten years and I am still working with him. It's funny how people outside our situation can see all the effort my recovery took, but it was very hard to get back on track with my family because they knew the Susana prior to all of this – especially my children – and they recognise that I don't have the same vigour I used to have. I have many ideas, but when it comes to putting them in place I don't have the energy, and my family cannot understand that.

I can be very slow at times and my children get annoyed if I don't do things at the speed they want – unless, of course, I experience hypomania and go to the other extreme. Then I might find myself out in the garden until 8.30 p.m. digging holes. I want to plant, so that's what I do. They think that's crazy. I do get an enormous amount of energy from time to time. But I am not the same.

Recently I was having breakfast with a friend from the support group. She is much younger than I am and first came to the group when she was depressed. 'Susana,' she asked me, 'how can I be like this? I've done so much with my life. I'm intelligent. I've got three degrees.' Make no mistake, she is a clever girl. This illness doesn't discriminate. She could easily sue her previous employers if she chose, as she had been given a terrible time and been seriously persecuted for her condition.

She understands her condition now but there was a time when she had refused to take any medication. On one occasion I had to insist that she go to the doctor. She did listen to me and now feels much better, although she still has regrets. She is grieving for all that she has lost.

I have also suffered loss. I lost the opportunity to finish my degree in America. I won a full scholarship. It was fully paid for, housing included, for four years in a beautiful college in Pennsylvania. And it was cut short to only four months. I could dwell on that, but where would that take me? Nowhere. So I have decided instead to accept it.

When I experienced the physical pain of depression, I did not want to wake up, day after day. Even when my head wanted me to get out of bed, my depression did not allow me. I realise that at this point I walked a thin line between life and death.

In May 2007, I lost my sister Silvia. We were very close. She committed suicide at 60 years of age, after being diagnosed with ovarian cancer. She was a highly intelligent person, an accountant, and knew exactly what she wanted and didn't want. After the diagnosis, she had the cancer removed and started chemotherapy. At that time she was very depressed and the chemotherapy made her feel worse. Silvia had a predisposition to depression, and after three suicide attempts she was admitted to a clinic. She was definite that she didn't want to live but then she started to get better, or so it seemed. Once she was released from the clinic she started doing well but, in truth, this was when she planned her suicide.

I decided to go to Argentina and see her in person as I couldn't stand only being able to talk to her on the telephone. She and her husband Eduardo came to the airport to welcome me. My mother and her husband were there too. We all went out for lunch, including my nephew, Jorge, whom we collected on the way to the restaurant. It was a lovely place, and during lunch Silvia made a toast. As we left, I kissed her goodbye and headed back to my mother's home.

The next day, Silvia jumped from the ninth floor of a building. She had planned the whole thing. That's why she had suddenly 'gotten better'. The lunch, the toast, were her way of saying goodbye. I wanted to spend time with her but she didn't give me the chance.

I believe that she had made up her mind and simply didn't want to change her plans.

I was not angry with my sister because I could understand her. In this case I didn't get the chance to tell her that the depression was responsible. But even if the depression had gone, the cancer would still have been there and she would eventually have died. My father also died from cancer.

This event did not affect my mental health because I had prepared for dealing with loss and grief. Before going to Argentina, I had attended a conference on suicide prevention, and the Salvation Army provided counselling for me on my return. I also had the support of my family.

I attended a healing program for my personal life, which I found very helpful. My husband was supportive of me attending this program and I am thankful for it, because it made me feel more confident and helped rebuild my self-esteem.

It can take two years after an episode for people with bipolar to get back on their feet. I try to help people distinguish between themselves and the depression. I often tell participants that the voice they hear is the depression speaking, not themselves. The support group is very good for me as my family get tired of hearing me talk about bipolar, but in the group it's OK to discuss it – people want to hear about it. They've been through it too and they understand. It is wonderful to not have to try and explain the unexplainable.

I also became a member of the Black Dog Institute steering committee. I attended conferences on bipolar disorder and diversity, and tried to educate myself and others through this organisation.

I am involved in projects with the Living Library. We are able to tell others about having bipolar disorder. I think education is very important in breaking down stigmas. The community should accept and treat mental illness as they would a physical illness.

My mother runs a nursing home in Argentina. A few years after the crisis had passed, unbeknown to me, she asked one of the visiting psychiatrists about bipolar disorder. He explained what it was and they discussed different medications and treatments. Some time after, I told her I wasn't feeling well and she suddenly suggested I should see my doctor about increasing my dosage of Effexor. I said, 'What?' I was stunned; I had no idea that she knew anything about bipolar, let alone Effexor. It was then that she began to take an active interest in how I was coping.

I am now fifty. Over the years I have learned to differentiate between sadness and bipolar depression. Receiving help and support from doctors, my husband, my family and therapy has helped me to develop the very positive way of thinking that I now have. I am grateful that I didn't die and am proud that I have accomplished a lot. I am finally enjoying myself! I do worry about my children, though. They are in their young adulthood, and this is the time that they may become vulnerable. I fear passing this illness onto my children.

The single most important message I have to pass on is a plea to those with mental health issues to continue taking your medication. Mental illness is not a game. It is a chemical imbalance in the brain. When you are given the right mix of chemicals to correct it, why wouldn't you take them? Should a diabetic refuse to take insulin? I tell people in my support group, and cannot emphasise this enough: if you have the right mix of medications that work for you, don't stop taking them. Be responsible for your health and wellbeing.

- If you believe bipolar is a chemical imbalance, then do not stop taking your medicine.
- If you are not happy with your doctor, do not hesitate to go to another. Trusting your doctor is very important – make sure you work as a team.
- Once you find structure in your day, try to follow it. Take things one day at a time. Only do as much as you want or can.
- Get friendly with your condition. Learn to know it as well

as possible, because the more you know it, the better you get along.

For me, education, true acceptance of the illness and a tailored maintenance program has given me a new life. Different – but still enjoyable.

Best wishes to you all for a healthy, happy and fulfilling life.

Five: Scarlett

A part of me died when I lost the ability to follow my dreams.

Not long ago, I heard someone say that how we deal with failure says more about us than whether or not we succeed. This is so very true: it was this thought that gave me the strength to find new dreams.

I believe that my symptoms of bipolar started early in my childhood. I look back on the small things and now recognise that often they weren't right.

I remember a particular homework assignment in grade three. We were told to write a list of ten words, each with four letters, that had the 'ea' sound. That night, I went through my giant Macquarie dictionary (note: all the other kids used children's dictionaries) and wrote out every single four-letter word with the 'ea' sound that I could find. The next day, my teacher walked around and checked off each child's homework. I will never forget the look of absolute shock on his face when he saw mine. I didn't understand his surprise though – it seemed the most natural thing in the world to find every single word. *All or nothing* could have been my mantra.

I did many similar things in primary school. I also endured waves of depression. At bedtime I longed not to live through the night. I often woke up in the mornings even sadder because I was still alive.

Dance, particularly ballet, was my passion from the very beginning. I had spectacular dreams and all the faith in the world that I could achieve them. I believed that all I had to do was work hard. I trained every day: on weekends, after school, all the time. But then, at around eleven years old, I started to experience panic attacks and fainting spells. I didn't understand what was happening and no one explained it to me. My mother didn't discuss it. My dance teacher tried to help but wasn't able to explain anything. Being so young, I just wanted someone to help and tell me what was going on.

My anxiety became more intense. One day, I was on stage performing a solo piece in a competition. I spun around, thoroughly enjoying being the centre of attention, but as my eyes met the audience I was instantly gripped by intense panic. I completely forgot what I was supposed to do next and ran off the stage in tears.

I didn't get a place although I did receive a wonderful write-up. I think that in the very moment when I lost my head, I also lost my self-confidence. I became depressed and comforted myself with food. Carrying even a few extra kilos is never a good thing for a dancer, so my teacher commented on it. I was already feeling down so I really took it personally, and felt particularly angry, as my dance teacher was considerably overweight herself. Starting puberty early didn't help. I was trying to manage a new chest size, periods and raging hormones. Now I was being told I was too fat.

I ended up leaving that dance school and going to another. Unfortunately, this place didn't offer the strict discipline that I craved. I left soon after joining and gave up on my dreams of ever becoming a dancer. It still hurts me to this day. I believe that if someone had reached out to me to help me through such a hard time in my life, things might have been different.

In high school, my anxiety and depression continued to gradually worsen. Many of my friends left school early, which was painful as it had been hard enough to make friends to begin with. Having to find more was even worse.

I was under a lot of pressure to choose Year 12 subjects. I had always been a straight-A student so everyone believed I wanted to go to university. It was too late for me to study ballet but I still wanted to go to the Academy of Performing Arts, so I chose subjects in art, music and graphic design. Many people were unhappy and disappointed in me for doing so.

This is when my struggle with depression really began. Although I am intelligent, I sat in an economics class and found myself unable to figure out basic equations. I spoke with the teacher and asked why I wasn't 'getting it'. She assured me that everything would soon fall into place; however, six months later nothing had, despite my continuous requests for help.

On the morning of my high school exams, I woke and wondered what the point was; I didn't understand any of it. So I lay in bed for the rest of the day and cried. I don't know why my mother didn't make me attend. She didn't even knock on the bedroom door throughout the day to see if I was all right.

My mother has passively watched me throughout my entire life. She has seen me fail, cry, succeed, become depressed, experience stress to the point of fainting and panic attack and has never done anything other than sit back and watch. I had reached quite a severe state of depression by this stage and I would shout at her repeatedly, 'Something is wrong, and you aren't helping me! Why aren't you helping me?' I felt so alone.

At the time, I felt that the only answer was to just go away; and my mother agreed. She organised a place for me to stay and within a couple of weeks I had moved to a small town on the coast on my own, intending to study Art and Design at TAFE. I spiralled further and further into depression, compounded by the fact that I was not old enough to drive a car and didn't have any friends. I spent my sixteenth birthday alone in my new room. It was so cold that the paper in my art books actually became wet and started to ripple. I felt so alone. By that night I had started to feel ill.

I became progressively worse and was eventually diagnosed with a severe case of glandular fever and had to return home to my parents. I had all the associated side-effects, including hepatitis, anaemia, some dysfunction of my liver and chronic fatigue. The fatigue was by far the worst. My eyes were too tired to even watch television. I just slept and slept. I wonder now whether I had glandular fever, or whether this had actually been some kind of breakdown.

Nearing recovery, I approached an old boss I had worked for in a supermarket and was given my previous job back. Things returned to how they were before I left. At work I met Mark who worked there as a baker, and soon I moved in with him . A few months after I turned seventeen, we made plans to move to Perth together. I applied for entry to several colleges to study in various fields of art and design, and was accepted into all of them. I chose Environmental Design.

Unfortunately, once I started, for reasons unknown to me at the time, I just couldn't 'get it together'. The teacher would ask us to complete a task, and within minutes my mind would be racing at a thousand miles an hour. I believed my work was sub-standard while everyone else's projects were brilliant. The panic would continue to escalate until I felt I had to escape. I would run away, and then become embarrassed about it and feel unable to return for up to two weeks at a time. On top of that, I then had to make up a story to explain why I hadn't been there.

On the very last day, students were required to show their creations. I worked tirelessly for three days and three nights, without sleep, to make up for a whole semester of not actually attending class. The time came and we publicly displayed our work in various forms. The lecturers, students and general public viewed my work but then something or someone set me off, and I fled. I waited for several hours until everyone had left, collected my compositions, threw them in the bin and raced home, never to be seen again. It turned out that I had actually won several awards and my work had been described as brilliant, but in my depression-induced tunnel vision, I was convinced that everyone was lying. I was relieved that my work would never again see the light of day. I asked my boss to turn my part-time job at the supermarket bakery into a full-time position and vowed to never to attempt art again.

I also realised that Mark and I weren't meant to be together and never really had been. He'd go out of his way to tell me that we'd never marry, even though I never sought to marry him. I'm sure I said things to him that were equally insensitive. He was only three years older than me but at that time, at that age, we were worlds apart. Mark would yell at me, telling me to get my shit together, and I would yell back at him to stop eating and spending hours on end on the game console.

I moved out and became very good friends with a wonderful girl from work, so I moved to a place nearer to her. I was earning a lot of money, had no real ties and no one to answer to. This marked the beginning of a very manic period of my life.

I ended up leaving my position for a job at a lunch bar. I also took on a second job, working in a restaurant at night. Even that wasn't enough so I found a third job, a casual catering position, to fill in any of the nights that I would have had free. Instead of going home after work, I would go out and party. I honestly don't know when I slept. Maybe I didn't!

I was a crazy party girl for a while, then I seemingly disappeared from the face of the earth. I assume people thought I wasn't interested in their lives, but the opposite was true. I was constantly thinking about them and wondering how to make contact. I know that I never did anything to be ashamed of, but in my mind, at the time, I believed that I could never show my face again. Anxiety and depression consumed me, until I cycled and became manic again.

The following year I felt drawn back to art. I found a wonderful graphic design course and enrolled. The first few weeks went smoothly but then the panic started again. It was so bad at times that I couldn't leave my house.

One of my depressive episodes went on for so long, I was convinced I must have had some kind of physical illness. I went to my local GP and told him I was having trouble sleeping, was struggling at the TAFE college and wasn't coping so well with life in general. The doctor started to talk to me about hormones and how it's common for girls my age to feel this way. I remember telling him that it just wasn't like me to be performing so poorly and he said, 'Well, you're just going to have to pull your socks up then, aren't you?' I left the surgery in tears.

I did have some good times, too. At one stage things were going well and I was attending college every single day until a bomb was dropped. My mother rang the college (rather than ringing my mobile) and asked one of the lecturers to tell me that she was leaving my father and that she was in a women's shelter. This news hit me like a hard punch to the stomach and brought me to my knees in the corridor. I was devastated. I went straight to her aid. She instructed me to immediately stop my studies, as I would have to support her from here on, and there would no longer be time or money for study. Of course, I was more than willing to do so but it never eventuated as my father came over, took her back home and nothing more was said. This wasn't the first or last time this happened.

I later realised that my mother had told people that my father had abused both her and me. She told me, when I was already in a state of depression, that all she'd known from my father was years of violence. This rocked me to the core. I had never seen or even suspected my father of being violent in any way to anyone. Eventually I realised that it wasn't true. I rang her, enraged, and she said that she had been referring to emotional violence.

I suddenly understood why I had been repeatedly dragged out of school by psychologists and social workers. I thought that was how life was. Dysfunctional was the norm.

One night I was feeling down and called my mother, who became hysterical and called the psychiatric hotline who in turn tried to call me. I had no intention of hurting myself. I was just very upset and couldn't understand why I couldn't hold down a job or study continuously, like a regular person.

During this time I met another guy. Andrew suited my manic personality to a tee. We were both hyperactive, spontaneous, 'stay out all night' kind of people. I later realised that he frequently used recreational drugs such as ecstasy. I had assumed he was on the same 'level' as me but, looking back now, I realise that although we were both 'high', his was the illegal variety.

I became very emotional. I would cry for no apparent reason and get very upset. I can understand that from Andrew's point of view, this would have been a very hard thing to deal with – a whole sudden change of personality – and Andrew had no compassion at all. Soon he told me it was too much drama to deal with. I was no longer 'fun'. We had only been together for a few months, and although it was an intense relationship, it was too much excitement for such a short space of time. He became very cold the moment I showed any 'weakness'.

He broke my heart. I see now, though, that the relationship was a short-term fit with my manic behaviour at the time. This relationship brought out the worst in me. I would've done anything for him. I turned into a weak, desperate woman. I was searching for that magical someone or something to make everything OK. I remained obsessed with him for a period of time afterwards. It was a very messed-up situation.

After many years I have realised the only thing that can make everything OK is self-acceptance, and that is something you can't buy. You must find it within.

I spent most of that year cycling between severe mania and depression. During one of my manic episodes – that lasted three weeks – I thought it suddenly important to do a bar course. I did not sleep for the entire duration of the course, which amazes me to this day. I was *the* personality of the class. Everyone adored me; at least I thought they did. But my steam ran out just as I was starting the fourth week and I never returned.

Eventually I swung again and picked up a job in the city waiting tables. I became paranoid. I thought deeply about everything that anyone said to me: much more than I should have. I was very focused on the fact that my boss couldn't remember my name and thought that meant I was doing a terrible job. One day he commented on the fact that my work shirt had stains on it so I went home, bleached my top (which was white) and fell to pieces when I realised the logo was also white: it should've been black. I ended up writing a crazy letter to my boss, ranting and raving about how he couldn't remember my name and announcing my resignation; then I suddenly became apologetic that he thought I had done a terrible job and suggested he keep my wages (which would have been substantial) because of the ruined shirt.

So again I endured waves of depression. Despite my previous negative experience with doctors I went to see another GP. I told him the same thing that I told the first doctor. He took my blood pressure and assured me if I lost weight, I would feel better. I was stunned.

A few months passed and my problems with panic attacks escalated. I drove to the Samaritans and met a lovely older lady who had the most calming voice. She told me that I was experiencing panic attacks. For so long I had believed that it was my fault. Discovering that there was actually something wrong with me was the best news I could have received. She gave me contact details for a psychologist who worked at a university and helped me work through my feelings.

At the end of that year I moved in with Ben, a friend of a friend, whom I'd kept in contact with. He is the funniest, most incredible and supportive person I've ever known. Just as I neared my twentieth birthday, my relationship with Ben moved to a different level and became stronger than ever. If it weren't for the support of Ben, the psychologist and my lecturers, I would never have completed my Diploma of Graphic Design.

Ben proudly came with me to my graduation event. He knew how hard this had been for me and took me out me to celebrate. For the first time in my life, someone truly loved me, was proud of me and really understood what I had been through.

Ben's work regularly took him away from home and he soon

suggested that I come with him. So off we went together and I found a great job with the local paper: my first graphic design position. I was only contracted to work three days a week, but I put in long hours to make sure everything was perfect. In keeping with my history, my brain stopped doing as it was told after a while and I started to make crucial mistakes. I started really falling apart.

I went to the mental health hospital after work every night, hoping that someone would help me. All the people with obvious extreme mental conditions who were threatening to stab others or set fire to themselves were admitted. By the time my turn came, it was closing time and I was told to come back the next day. I did this every night for about three weeks. I remember musing that I should run in with a fake weapon of some kind so I would receive help more quickly. I didn't dare ring my mother, as I knew I would not get any support and would end up feeling worse – and guilty for feeling how I was.

I was eventually told that I had depression. This really surprised me, because I had thought depression was something that only affected old people. I left in a daze. I told Ben about the diagnosis and I knew it was time to return home. It was hard, as he still had to work away. I would hardly ever see him as his 'fly in, fly out' schedule required six weeks away for every one week at home.

Previously, while I was studying Graphic Design, our lecturers had instructed us to create postcards. They were brief resumes with some fantastic eye-catching design to help us secure jobs. I still had plenty left over, so while making arrangements to return home, I sent out the postcards to potential employers. I ended up sending them to every single design house I could find in the phonebook, but that's bipolar for you!

Even before I returned home I was accepted for quite a few interviews and I landed a fantastic position at a massive printing house. Life was going well again. I was being paid well, I had bought a nice car, and again I was working many long hours, far more than was required. I wanted to impress my boss and it paid off. Clients began asking for me by name. To be in demand in this way, at the age of 21, with barely any experience, earned me a lot of respect.

But again, I pushed myself too hard. My poor brain overloaded and the panic returned. I started making mistakes. It seems as though I just switched off and operated on some kind of auto-pilot, faxing proofs to random numbers and emailing clients for details they had already given me.

One day while having coffee with a friend, she confided that she was having the same kind of problems and was seeing a psychiatrist. I managed to obtain a referral, but the waiting list was a joke. I was literally unravelling and had no time to waste. I repeatedly tried to see the psychiatrist, in complete desperation, as I believed that he was the only person in the entire world who could help me. The nurse at his surgery took me aside in the office one day as all I could do was cry and rock myself, saying, 'Why won't anyone help me?' over and over. She had a terrible look on her face, like her heart was breaking, but I was once again sent home.

I finally saw the psychiatrist and was given medications. I tried various antidepressants for about six months before I realised that the times I believed I had been going well were actually manic episodes. That came as a great disappointment to me as I really thought that I was getting better.

At the age of 21 I was diagnosed by my psychiatrist as having bipolar disorder. That day I was extremely upset about the diagnosis, but ended up on a bit of a high afterwards. The high gave me the confidence to tell my boss that I was sick and I needed some time away from work to heal. I joked that the bottle of water I carried around everywhere (as my medication made me thirsty) was really straight vodka. He laughed. He was pleased to have an explanation for why I had been on fire one minute and almost useless the next. I only told him that I had depression. I believed I would need a few months to recuperate and would be back. Little did I know I had started the fight of my life.

I didn't tell my boss that I had bipolar disorder because at the time I believed that depression was curable but bipolar affects your behaviour for your entire life. Of course that's not true, but I didn't realise this at the time.

I called my mother to let her know that I had quit my job. What a mistake that was. Instead of supporting me, she became completely hysterical and shrieked at me over the phone, saying that she couldn't be expected to take care of me financially. This was not the response that I needed. I was in a stable relationship and financially fine, with a home shared by my partner. I was only calling for the emotional support any daughter would normally expect to receive from her mother.

Things were rough for a while. I had my friend who, freakishly, had been diagnosed with bipolar disorder just a month before. We became much closer friends and really helped each other through those times. Sometimes we would just sit in silence for hours. It was comfortable and lovely.

I told other friends about my diagnosis around six months later. Some asked questions and others hadn't a clue. I was tired of lying to people and saying, 'Oh, I think I have a cold coming on,' so without getting heavy, and only if needed, I decided to just let people know if I wasn't doing so well and that I was taking a break.

In late November in 2004, I had a sudden driving urge to be 'clean' though I wasn't manic at the time. I immediately stopped my medication and changed my diet. I stopped drinking alcohol, taking any drugs and started eating lots of fresh fruit and vegetables. I had been taking 80mg of Aropax (Paxil), 800mg of Lithium and 2000mg of Epilium every day and I stopped taking them all just like that. Cold turkey.

A couple of weeks later I realised my period was late but I didn't want to think about what that might mean. I just kept on living my 'clean' lifestyle. A couple of weeks later again, my period still hadn't come and I knew that it was time to deal with the situation. I purchased two pregnancy test kits and they both came out positive. I cried my heart out in Ben's arms because I thought I might be forced to have an abortion: my psychiatrist had told me it was extremely dangerous to be on Epilium while pregnant.

My psychiatrist was very upset with me. It turned out that my 'clean' urge had given my baby a much better chance, as I had only taken Epilium for two weeks or so since conception. My psychiatrist made me feel guilty for getting pregnant and pushed me to have an abortion. She insisted that I was in no state to look after a child. By having a baby, I would probably relapse and have major problems with breastfeeding.

She sent me to another psychiatrist for a second opinion. He was an incredibly calm and patient man, and even though things didn't look good, he told me the truth. I was going to need many ultrasounds and could choose to have an abortion before twelve weeks if the foetus showed major health problems such as a lack of brain growth or spina bifida. I also had a further option to abort before twenty weeks, but that would require an induction. I found the thought of this truly horrific.

I went for regular ultrasounds and everything looked good each time. I continued to hope but I dared not buy anything baby-related. I tried to pretend it wasn't really happening in case I did have to abort: maybe then it would hurt less.

To our great relief and joy, after the twenty-week scan we were able to celebrate the fact that our baby had a good chance of being born healthy. And he was.

The day after his birth, the midwife showed me how to make formula – I had chosen not to breastfeed – and I found I just couldn't take it in. I simply couldn't understand. She reassured me and said that it was due to tiredness. I had a bad feeling about it but tried to convince myself that she was right.

Later that day, I was given some medication for my back – I had strained it during childbirth – and I had a sudden, allergic reaction to the medication. I also started to 'wig out'. I became so itchy, anxious and panicked that I wanted to run out of the hospital, into the night.

I felt close to one of the midwives and I thank God that she came into the room at just the right moment. I told Ben to take the baby to the lounge. I grabbed the midwife and told her I believed I was having some kind of manic reaction and I needed something to help me NOW! I wedged myself between a machine attached to the wall and my bed, hoping that that would help me stay in the hospital.

The midwife calmly sat on my bed and talked to me. I couldn't stop moving, talking and frantically looking around. Everything was going so fast. It was the worst panic attack of my life. After what felt like a very long time I was given some Valium under the tongue and other anti-psychotics. When the drugs took effect, I eventually fell asleep. That was the closest I've ever felt to 'crazy' and I never want to be there again.

The next day my psychiatrist came to see me. Usually he was warm and comfortable to talk to but this time he wasn't. He just stood at the end of my bed holding a clipboard. I felt like a freak. I was prescribed anti-psychotics during the day with a large dose in the evening. Ben was asked to stay at the hospital and look after our baby during the night. It was a terrible time for him and I feel incredibly guilty for putting him through it.

We were allowed to go home ten days later. That's when the depression kicked in.

I was told to take our baby to a place that helps new mums learn how to feed and bond with their baby. The thing was, this wasn't my problem. I had it all organised. Feeding times, how to change his nappy, the 'mechanics' of taking care of baby were no problem. It was my sadness that wasn't OK. They made me talk about my life, which I found to be a painful ordeal. They asked why I was sad and I told them straight out: 'I am upset because I have postnatal depression, so I have to take my antidepressants and ride out the wave.' But they continued asking me questions. Talking to some people about depression is like trying to convince a racist to respect people who aren't the same colour. There's no point.

They told me I was feeding my baby too much although the midwives from the hospital had told me it was excellent and that my son was feeding well. I became angry and told them I would be leaving in the morning. It is so unhelpful to pick someone apart who is suffering so much. It is actually quite dangerous. I only stayed there for one night.

The next twelve months were a lonely time for me. I felt unable to talk to anyone else but Ben. Every now and then I tried, but most people didn't understand. I remember trying to talk to a friend about my feelings of despair. She looked at me blankly and asked, 'But don't you love your baby?'

People simple cannot fathom how you can have a baby and not feel overwhelming love for it, the very first moment you hold it. Having a baby equalled pain to me. Not physical pain, but endless emotional pain. Pain that seemed like it would never stop. I felt as though the baby had sucked everything out of me and gave nothing back but dirty nappies. I felt as though having the baby had put an end to my life.

But of course, the problem was never the baby. If my son ever reads this account, I hope he can understand:

> The problem wasn't you. It was never you. It was me and how I felt about babies, about life, and about myself. I thought having a baby was the end and that there would never be any time for me, ever again. But now I see what a miracle you truly are. You made me realise that it isn't just about me. You have shown me what a wonderful world it is. You lead me to find joy in simple things like bubbles floating in the air, splashing water, riding the escalators up and down (many times!) and eating ice cream. You haven't stopped my life, you have improved it a million-fold and without you, I wouldn't be the person I am today.

I look back at the behaviours I learnt from my mother. After hearing on a daily basis that I ruined her life and stopped her from living, it's no surprise that I thought having a baby was the end. Her favourite line (suitable for use in the soap operas that she loves so much) was, 'I sacrificed my life for you!'

It's not an excuse but I have realised how ingrained these messages became. And you can't stop something if you can't recognise it.

I did feel grateful, in a way, that I had already experienced depression. So I knew that eventually the engulfing darkness would subside. Yet it still hurt so much. I remember going to parties and gatherings together with my son. I would often end up sitting in the car and just crying. My heart – my soul – ached so much. I tried to tell myself that it would be over soon, but it was no comfort. It's a hard task, escaping depression.

I felt that I was trapped inside a bubble. The things that might have actually made me feel good escaped my mind. Eventually, when my son was around six months old, I got into the habit of lying on the grass in the sun by the river while my son crawled around me and later learned to walk. I believe that the simple act of doing this a few times a week was the beginning of my recovery. It was as if the sunlight started literally warming my soul.

I have reached a turning point in my life. I recently got married; and as lovely as that was, people behaved in strange ways in the lead-up to, and during, the wedding. That put quite a dent in my rose-coloured glasses.

I'm also sad to say that there are people I have looked up to and admired, believing they were resilient, confident people, and I have now realised that they aren't so strong. As my friends go though life and battle everyday things I see some of them beginning to unravel. This has made me realise that I'm not as weak as I thought I was. I do have great personal strength. I also realise that I should not be ashamed of my likes and dislikes, be they dress sense, sexual preferences or friendships that I have.

I also believe that my father has undiagnosed bipolar disorder, although he disagrees. My father self-medicates with antidepressants at times, which send him manic after a few days. In his mind, he's 'fixed' till he cycles into depression again.

When I was a child, my father was fun. I thought he was trying to keep my mother at bay when he joked about her wild stories. My mother would always say, 'Don't tell your father,' about the simplest of things; but we still maintained a bond. In the end, though, he is an enabler of her behaviour.

I now attribute much of the 'fun' approach to his manic behaviour. When in a manic state, my father doesn't respect rules or discipline. He will let my child draw on the walls while I'm in another room, and will talk to my son while he's in the 'naughty chair' and shouldn't be talking to anyone. His behaviour leads me to believe he has no respect for me as a parent or a person.

However, I am breaking free. I have realised that my mother has chosen to act like this and it is no reflection on my character. She chose to have a child, and though she clearly struggles with her own issues, it is wrong for me to feel guilty for my existence. I have found the strength and courage to move on and we are no longer in contact. Unfortunately, I am no longer in contact with my father either as he has chosen to side with my mother.

One of my key difficulties has always been constant worry about what other people think of me and whether my decisions are right, even when I'm sure they are. My wedding gave me a breakthrough realisation about how much energy I spend on trying to please other people. The truth is that you can never please everyone, sometimes not even one person. As long as you're happy and remain true to yourself, that's all you can do. In the past I have seemed to let life carry me along and take me for a ride, but now it's my turn to take control.

I have kept a solid relationship with my husband for eight years.

For a good part of our relationship he worked away from home, but he was recently promoted and now works closer by. My son attends family day care once a week to give me a chance to unwind and take care of errands and appointments.

Seeing a psychologist has been the most healthful strategy for me. In my experience I find psychiatrists are more focused on medication. Each session with a psychiatrist (and I've had about six different psychiatrists) follows the same routine. I tell them what's been happening and they adjust my dose accordingly. It's not fair to generalise, but it's my experience that many of them didn't look into why I was feeling a certain way before upping my dose. Sometimes there are reasons for feelings that can be helped by a good chat.

I have now been off medications, apart from the occasional Xanax for anxiety, since June 2006. I have been stable for over three years. Although I would never recommend that people with bipolar disorder go without medication, I suggest you find someone who does understand, is willing to help you and respects the fact that medication is not the only treatment for bipolar disorder.

I still have small mood swings. They don't happen often, but when they do I am able to control them. They can be triggered by having too much coffee and staying up too late.

I am a mother so I need to be responsible: I am quick to get on top of things. I will take medication if I need to – I just prefer not to unless absolutely necessary. I have achieved wellness through:

- Routine, routine, routine. I have a diary to record times, activities, appointments and (countless) lists.
- Exercise: it is essential for me to find my centre.
- Diet: sugary food and junk food are extremely bad for my moods. The extent to which diet affects me is truly amazing so I aim for low GI foods and small meals more often. This has also helped me with weight loss, so it's a double bonus!
- Spending time with my son. He shows me the beauty in the simple things in life.

- Not putting extra pressure on myself when I'm feeling stressed. I am kinder to myself now. I try to adopt an attitude of doing my very best at the time rather than the frustrating and frequently disappointing 'all or nothing' approach!
- Minimising coffee intake. And I never drink it after 3 p.m.
- Sleep is crucial, at the appropriate times.
- Talking: I talk to shrinks, psychologists, good friends, anyone! I have made such great strides since I started seeing a psychologist. I talk and set goals. I am currently working towards my goal of owning a successful online business.
- I don't let things build up and I acknowledge the validity of my feelings.

The next chapter in my life will involve our second child. I am currently in the very early stages of my second pregnancy. Having my first child was quite an ordeal but I am now ready. I'm going to ask every question and talk to everyone I possibly can, because good information is what I deserve. I refuse to be afraid.

I have bipolar disorder but I consider myself in remission. I only experience relapses when my life goes out of balance. Of course my life is not always in perfect balance, but regaining this is a big key for me. Not working endless hours at my job, not working out at the gym till I haven't got time for anything else. No endless partying, or being a Mum full time with no down time at all. It's all about balance. A little bit of everything.

If you have, or think you have bipolar disorder, I encourage you to read, listen, talk and use any source you can to learn about it. Knowledge really is power. If you're not happy with your situation, find the answers you need.

It's one of the hardest things to do, but don't stop until you find a mental health practitioner that you're happy with, whether a psychiatrist, a psychologist or a general practitioner.

My journey so far has also taught me not to be ashamed of who I am. So what if I'm more sensitive than other people? I can also be an incredible tower of strength. So what if I'm grumpy and emotional if I've had a bad night's sleep? When well rested I can generate fantastic ideas and creations. This is who I am! As long as I am responsible and don't let my highs and lows affect my relationships with friends and my family, I will embrace who I am.

Although I can't claim to be in total control, I have one firm hand on the steering wheel. As I begin to stand up for myself, I know I must deal with criticism. However, I know what is best for me and for my son. My instinct, particularly where it relates to my son and his health, is never wrong. I am starting to listen to myself. I trust me.

I am beginning to know who I am and what I like. I am unique and I embrace my individuality. I am no longer ashamed to be different.

If you ever lose your dreams, dare to dream again.

Six: Ciara

I was born to Scottish parents and had a boisterous, enjoyable, artistic and free childhood. There were many parties and much singing in our household, particularly from my father and grandfather. I enjoy close relationships with most of my siblings and I am now also close to their children.

In primary school I was a diligent student and got along well with both teachers and classmates. I was almost every teacher's pet. However, high school was a different story. Some children just don't make the transition from primary to high school smoothly and I was one of them. I had left a close community at primary school and joined a much larger, more impersonal environment. I became very disruptive in class. I didn't want to 'play up' but felt I couldn't help it. I spoke out of turn and would simply get up out of my seat if I felt like it.

Because of my poor behaviour, I was excluded from classes on two occasions but, surprisingly, my parents were never contacted. I don't think the school had much of a behaviour management policy at that time, and the teachers probably didn't know how to handle me. Except for my art teacher. Most teachers would scream and yell but my art teacher was firm and fair. She was able to reach me. On one occasion she looked at me and said, 'You've got a good family and you've got a good brain. Don't just waste your chances!' I really took that on board. She became a close friend for a number of years after I finished school.

I didn't know what I wanted to do when I left school. During Year Eleven, I wanted to be a back-up singer, as I had a good voice until I came down with a bout of the flu.

I continued to sing despite the flu but found that when the virus left me, my singing voice went with it.

I didn't have any close friends in high school until my matriculation year in 1982. No career counselling was offered and, given how I had behaved, I think the staff just wanted me to leave as quickly as possible. As a result, and out of habit, I had chosen matriculation subjects that I didn't like, such as maths and chemistry, and failed the exams. Over the following summer I grew up a little, settled down and returned to school in 1983, selecting humanities subjects that I enjoyed. That year I passed matriculation with good grades.

Between failing and starting Year Twelve again, I realised that I had to drastically change the way I was living my life. My misbehaviour had been extreme by any standards and I was perturbed by it, even as it occurred. After some serious reflection, I went on to university study in 1984, a well-contained and well-adjusted individual.

I had yet to have an episode of illness I could clearly identify as an indicator of bipolar disorder, but I had begun to experience signs of light-headedness around the age of twenty, during those hectic university years.

I studied drama as part of my degree and was chosen to be the stage manager for the year's student performance. I thrived on the close contact with so many students and decided to help out at the University Theatre Guild as stage manager, and the University Dramatic Society as touring manager. The combined student and volunteer workload amounted to around seventy hours of pressure each week, but I loved it and decided that I wanted to work in the entertainment industry, both creatively and behind the scenes.

I graduated in 1987. I excelled in the part-time job at a department store that saw me through university, gaining many customer commendations. I oversaw a small department within menswear, where I made some good friendships with fellow sales assistants and was respected by management.

At the age of 22, I had a breakdown after completing two 'rebirthing' or 'clearing' workshops. These sessions were intense emotional experiences, and it was probably my participation that triggered the serious symptoms of my underlying bipolar condition.

It was stocktake time at the department store and I found myself unable to count properly as I worked on the merchandise sheets. I went downhill quickly. I found it difficult to concentrate and was even unable to string words together to have a conversation at times. I gave up the job. I began to feel less and less solid, as if I was losing control of my thoughts and my life in general. My thinking was disjointed and I struggled to make decisions and choices. The confusion and depression became so intense that I could barely speak at all, and later that year I even found it a challenge to walk. I once heard Irish singer Sinead O'Connor say on the Oprah show that wellness feels like a solid brick wall while falling ill with bipolar disorder feels as though the wall is falling apart, brick by brick. This describes well what an episode has felt like for me. For most of 1988, I didn't eat or drink properly because my thinking was so fuzzy that I was distracted by the psychological pain and was simply not aware that I needed sustenance.

A friend of mine, my former art teacher, had visited a psychic in earlier years, and suggested that I do the same. That visit led me to develop an interest in channelling. I travelled to the United States for one month, to attend a channelling workshop. I went on my own and shared accommodation with other workshop attendees.

The leader of the group recommended a breathing technique which was said to open one's brain to receive greater knowledge. After using the technique for an extended period during the course of the workshop, I had a near-death experience. I believe that the experience occurred because I was unwell at the time. My body had reached its limits and was beginning to shut down. I had dropped two dress sizes and had become very thin.

After the near-death experience I felt very bad indeed. I had no goals. I became fuzzier in my thinking and generally felt as if I'd been hit by a bus! Thankfully, I had become aware that something was wrong with me and began eating properly again. I became more aware of how I felt.

Once I was back in Australia, my family took me to see a general practitioner and I was referred to a psychiatrist. I was very depressed at the time and not able to communicate effectively with others, though I had previously been articulate.

I made a half-hearted attempt to take my life in 1989 because of physical pain which was possibly due to the side-effects of my medication. I didn't want to die but I sought peace and believed that if I died I'd be with Jesus and everything would be OK.

My belief system at the time included investigating the concept that we might be considered gods because we can create aspects of our lives. This was a belief considered by many people I knew, particularly friends who were involved in New Age practices. After telling my first psychiatrist this, she incorrectly diagnosed me as having schizophrenia.

I can understand why the doctor made this diagnosis; however, she did not explore the conventional aspects of my life in assessing me. She asked if I heard voices or thought that the television station was broadcasting just for me. I didn't have either of these symptoms. I was given a particular antipsychotic drug and became even more depressed while taking it. I also gained a huge amount of weight.

My second psychiatrist was a wonderful person and prescribed a different drug, which seemed to control any highs but produced side-effects of restlessness and muscle stiffness. I took it for some months before becoming unwell again, leading to my first hospitalisation after a Reiki course. My parents were interstate and my doctor didn't know I had private health insurance, so my first hospitalisation, in

1992, was in the public health system. The environment was very challenging. Fellow patients were very unwell and I often felt they weren't properly attended to. Some people were violent and had frequent outbursts. It was really frightening.

During this time, I couldn't hold down a job and lost contact with most of my friends because I couldn't communicate effectively. My independence was reduced and the friendships I did manage to keep were often unequal. I was somewhat subservient, so my trust was sometimes abused.

I was hospitalised again in the following year and experienced great fear to begin with, given my previous experience in the public system. This time, however, I entered the private health system and it was a different experience.

I was hospitalised twice in 1994, once after undertaking a sweat lodge. This is a North American Indian religious ceremony that takes place in a tent-like structure.

Hot rocks are placed in the middle, and it's similar to a sauna. It is a purification ritual during which people pray and set intentions. I became dehydrated during one of these ceremonies, and this triggered an episode that resulted in hospitalisation for around three weeks. I later spoke with a North American Indian woman who told me that people who are not of North American Indian descent should not undertake these sacred ceremonies. I never did so again.

During the early 1990s I did volunteer work, when I was able, at the Women's and Children's Hospital and the State Theatre shop. I was a volunteer during the Third International Women Playwrights Conference, and performed with a visiting South Korean shaman. This amazing woman, Kim Kum Hwa, granted me an audience and I felt comfortable enough to tell her about my health experiences. She told me that in her country, such experiences occur regularly in young adulthood as part of a shamanic awakening.

In 1995, my friend and former art teacher passed away. So, for a retreat, I joined a community of Buddhist monks and resided there for five months. It was a public meeting place for Mahayana Buddhists. I shared accommodation with two Tibetan, one Nepalese and one Australian monk.

At the age of thirty, I was again admitted to hospital in a 'high state' and was correctly diagnosed with bipolar disorder by my current psychiatrist.

There was a feeling of fear within my family when I was originally diagnosed with schizophrenia, and they expressed considerable relief when it was discovered that I 'only' had bipolar disorder. There was little, if any, discussion about bipolar disorder within my family. That suited me well because I wanted to minimise the effect it had on my life.

I decided to move on and become as healthy as I can. Talking with my doctors is enough, with the occasional brief explanation to people if I am feeling unwell.

I did share my diagnosis and some symptoms with friends, and as a result I lost most of the relationships. After losing these friendships, I decided to be more assertive and accept more of what I want in all relationships. I still wish to be easygoing and a soft place for people to fall, but I want to feel equal as well. I placed others on a pedestal too often and some of my past friendships reflected that. I understand that some old friends were afraid of my condition, so they backed away from me. That was their right.

My last hospitalisation was in 1996. Since then, I have been more aware of my thinking and can see that catastrophising about anything for too long may lead to an episode.

Before the illness presented in me, I had a very strong mind and true grit, and I still do. I became fed up with feeling unwell, so somewhere in this process, I began to love myself again.

In 1999, I heard of Cognitive Behavioural Therapy (CBT). My doctor gave me a referral to a ten-week course at a therapy centre. I enjoyed learning techniques and gaining tools which still assist me today to challenge and change my thinking whenever it is not useful.

CBT helps me to sort the wheat from the chaff, to lighten up and to realise that reality can be relative.

If I change the way I view a situation, I can decrease the intensity of the uncomfortable and unhappy emotions I sometimes feel. This greatly reduces the load on my emotional brain, and less stress means less chance of a breakdown.

I have managed my health with CBT techniques, appropriate medication, increasing maturity and awareness, and with great support from doctors, counsellors and therapists.

I have developed the confidence to intercept that feeling of slipping into a high, and am learning to *think my way well* again. To do this, I stop, slow everything down physically and mentally and remember that I have been here before and that I have recovered. My psychiatrist has given me permission to increase my medication by a small amount in such an instance, as long as I ring him within 24 hours to let him know. After several days on an increased dosage, I am usually feeling a lot better and more 'solid'. I have averted some potentially major episodes this way.

I am becoming an empowered, loving individual once more. I feel more secure within myself because I believe in my abilities to relate to people and demonstrate my empathy by listening to others and showing I care. I am less insular when well. I have always been optimistic, except when depressed in my teenage years, and I am nearly always hopeful, for both myself and others.

I can't overemphasise the need to have a doctor or therapist whom you trust and feel comfortable with. Healthy therapeutic relationships are important to healing and they have helped me to mature. I have also received great support from a homeopath, and believe people are well served by having health care options.

In 2000 I returned to university and studied towards a graduate education degree. Loving the social justice slant of the courses, I did well academically and received Distinctions or High Distinctions for most assignments and courses. I was also awarded a Sir Charles Bright Scholarship, for students with a disability, in 2003.

I have been single for most of my adult life. I might have remained single even if I didn't have bipolar disorder, because I possibly don't need a romantic relationship. I love the freedom of being single while realising that if I was in a healthy romantic relationship, there would be different kinds of freedom. I get along very well with men, in general, and love their company. Anyone I would choose to enter a romantic relationship with would be a kind and understanding person, so I don't have any real fears that I would be rejected because of bipolar disorder.

I would guide a man through my illness if I wished to take up any opportunity for a relationship. There is no reason why I couldn't have a partner one day. However, if I remain single, my life will still be great.

I would have loved to have children. I feel that having children is a privilege, not a right, and that children are, as Kahlil Gibran wrote in *The Prophet*, 'life's great longing for itself'. We do not own children – we are here to guide them. I have been privileged to help friends and family raise their children. I have had little time to regret that I am not a mother. Life is too beautiful to have regrets.

I could be interested in finding some more close friendships, though. There is distance between myself and old friends who live interstate or far away. I'd like some new friends, particularly now that I am in my mid-forties and life is changing again.

I am finding greater serenity and I am ready to have equal relationships. I practise love and understanding in all of my relationships, and, all in all, have a wonderful life.

If I had remained well during my adult years, I probably would have obtained more tertiary qualifications than I have. I am interested in psychology and social sciences, particularly social justice issues. I have an interest in Aboriginal education and special education. I might have liked to work with children with autism or children with behavioural difficulties. Freelance journalism also holds some interest.

Unfortunately, I have found it very stressful to study in recent years. Once again, I have no real regrets. I am learning to work with the health I have. For years I wanted to work in theatre and entertainment. Unfortunately, such work is high-pressure. Once again, no regrets. I now intend to explore different forms of writing, as this is both relaxing and exciting for me.

Over the past eleven years, I have compiled a collection of poetry on love, nature, the spirit and healing. Those English lessons at school and university have paid off! I have recently had the writing professionally assessed as publishable; so I will now revise my work and look for an illustrator. I generally write only when inspired to do so. Even though I have experienced heavy depressions and highs, my writing is still light in nature. It is not regular work, but is very meaningful for me. It uplifts me and inspires me to be part of life. Life is spectacularly worthwhile.

A great achievement I have made is to begin to accept my health condition, and, for many years now, to love and respect myself in the face of every adversity. Acceptance is the key, and realistic and hopeful living the result.

Self-awareness and the observation of my thoughts are solid achievements which prevent major relapses. I believe it is realistic to seek full or partial recovery. I have achieved the latter and manage bipolar symptoms daily.

I had a well-formed, healthy personality and character before I became seriously unwell; and I still do. I had a very happy and contented childhood, and this has been a vital platform for the recovery I've made. I have experienced some loss of confidence due to the bipolar condition, but sense that this too is beginning to turn around. I feel a new sense of confidence as I choose to overcome anxiety, using CBT techniques and my own self-respect and will.

I have felt a bit embarrassed at times about having bipolar

disorder, but I have come to realise that many people have some form of health challenge and bipolar disorder should be viewed as just that – a health challenge, not a character flaw. I am learning to feel equal to others again.

I am essentially more confident now than before I first experienced an episode of bipolar disorder because I have consciously chosen to continue to grow and mature. I have needed to focus less on New Age philosophies and more on traditional belief systems, such as Christianity and Buddhism, and have gained benefit from their tools for living a good life. My current psychiatrist believes that New Age practices have led to an increased incidence of mental illness among the population over the past twenty years. In my case, they tend to take me into an unhealthy 'high' state.

I am currently reassessing my belief system, and hope to have the greatest faith in myself and my ability to overcome adversity. My study of Jesus and the Buddha, both as a child and an adult, has helped me to take responsibility for my life, and to feel more worthy of my own love and respect. I am Christian but not interested in dogma. I am not interested in the politics of religion.

The first effective strategy I used to climb away from depression and confusion was to accept that I am both loving and lovable. When I felt worthy of my own love and support, I began to take small steps towards healing. For a while, I looked up at the sky each day and was amazed by its beauty and enduring quality. The sky held a real 'wow' factor for me. Even the act of looking upwards was helpful. Nature is always helpful to healing, because it doesn't judge and it doesn't rush.

Other strategies I use include:

- Losing the weight I had piled on due to medication side-effects. I made a motivational tape of my favourite pop music, got on the exercise bike and rode ten miles every day. I made myself walk around the neighbourhood too, and this expanded my mind to include others, and life, again.
- Humour: I rely on humour to lift me up, daily. I aim to be as

light-hearted as possible. Fortunately, having this condition has enabled me to put everyday woes into perspective; some things don't really matter to me anymore, though I still care about the struggles of others.

- I am in the process of accepting myself completely and this will be a solid platform for further healing. By sharing my thoughts for inclusion in *Inspired Recovery,* I feel a warm glow and optimism.

- Cognitive Behavioural Therapy (CBT) has assisted me enormously. I have completed two courses, each with a different structure and approach, and was able to integrate both, taking from each what works best for me.

- A great relationship with my doctor, and appropriate medication. Having been misdiagnosed for about seven years, I really appreciate the correct treatment and a healthy therapeutic relationship.

- Healthy, realistic thinking is vital to my staying well. When I start to ruminate over something that is bothering me, I now tell myself to stop, slow down and look at the underlying issues. I sometimes end up having a bit of a laugh at myself, and it is fascinating to see how far I have come in creating a healthy thinking process.

I experience more joy, calm, peace of mind, happier relationships and a willingness to participate because I am more confident about being able to communicate. I am cultivating a belief that I am eternal, and that my true nature cannot be harmed. A belief that reincarnation could be a reality gives me peace of mind that I have more opportunities to work out situations that sometimes trouble me, such as confusion in relationships.

To manage my condition, I have 'one days', 'two days' and 'three days', where I decide early on in the day how many things I can reasonably achieve without harming my health. Sometimes the 'one day' has been a day when I have needed to complete an assignment for a university course, or it might be doing the laundry – or even just making my meals, if I am not feeling too well on that day. Always on the agenda is to live consciously and to find as much enjoyment in the day as possible.

I am becoming gentle with myself, forgiving myself for putting myself through this, and conversely congratulating myself for putting myself through the process of having this condition. It has all been for purposeful good. I can now understand the plight of others more deeply. Once you've suffered, you can transfer that learning to empathy for the pain of others and the joy of others.

It brings me great fulfilment to see how far I have come from being stuck in a desperately depressive state in years past. Hoping that I can contribute usefully to others' lives brings me solace.

I encourage anyone suffering from mental illness to:

- Act as early as possible to intercept troubling thoughts; then you will find healing much easier. Focus on problem-solving as soon as possible to avoid getting stuck in a mental rut.

- Try to see the situation as just that – a situation – a neutral happening that is neither good nor bad. I know this is a big challenge; yet wisdom can be gleaned from this illness, so don't always wish it away; instead embrace it, acknowledge it and accept it. In doing this you will learn from the situation and be better able to move on.

- Don't judge your situation as bad, or your frame of reference will cause you to see more bad in your experience, and in the world. The eyes do not see, the brain does; and when we focus on unpleasant situations or sensations, such perceptions can eventually be wired into the brain itself, causing us to 'see' more unpleasantness in our lives, the lives of others, and in the world.

- Have a healthy focus; it is vital to healing. I recently learnt that the brain can be 'plastic' and that unfavourable brain changes can possibly be reversed. It is important to be aware of one's thinking, though. How we think and feel affects our brain's development.

- Take as much responsibility for your health as you can. Do all that you can for yourself – it is good for your self-esteem and motivation. Let others help you, but try not to become too physically, emotionally or mentally dependent on others. Healthy independence can translate into more thorough healing.

- Don't allow patronising behaviour you may receive from some medical staff, case workers, family, friends or anyone at all to lead you to believe that this reflects your worth. Recognise when their behaviour stems from their own fear or inability to cope with your situation. Be assertive but not reactive. Sometimes turning the other cheek – and having compassion for the ignorance of others – is appropriate and safer for you if you're in hospital under supervision.

- Have a long-term plan to heal and be patient with yourself. Leave room in your thinking for great healings to occur and don't believe that your condition is necessarily permanent. Some people experience a full recovery. Have a hopeful attitude. Because I am responsible, I will say that I hope to heal further, but use medication and my wise doctor's advice.

- Have gratitude for everything. It's all food for thought, and for your personal evolution.

- Give yourself love and attention; try not to seek too much of it from others. Plug up all your emotional holes. We all have to do this, whether we have health challenges or not. Be the source of your own fulfilment.

- Cultivate an observant nature. Observe your thoughts, without judgment. The more readily you can detect any unfavourable changes in your thinking and in your emotional states, the sooner you can rectify your attitudes and thought patterns and return to a healthy mind state. Observe people who do not have clinical mental health challenges, and see that they sometimes struggle as well. We are not alone.

- Try Cognitive Behavioural Therapy and apply it consistently. It does work. Effort and belief in both yourself and your therapist are important. It is a skill set that would benefit anyone, well or otherwise, and it is a portable skill set that can benefit you for life. Once rehearsed and practised, it remains part of your makeup and can create a wonderful view of the world.

- Work to have healthy self-talk. Challenge unhelpful thinking and replace it with healthy self-talk. Healthy self-belief is paramount to becoming and remaining well. If we value ourselves, we tend to behave in ways that promote our wellbeing.

- Surrender and accept what you cannot change, and be willing to do something about what you can change for the better. I suspect that everyone's health might be improved by a change in attitude – the attitude to one's self, and to life in general.

- Avoid sugar and caffeine. I have found that too much of either can make me feel less solid and a bit too jittery, for too long.

- Avoid alcohol. It is a depressant and usually doesn't work well with medications.

- Try to remain as light-hearted as possible. English writer G K Chesterton said, 'Angels fly because they take themselves so lightly.'

- Actively seek happy experiences. A Christian minister I knew used to say that people don't necessarily become dejected because so many bad things happen to them – it is because so few good things happen in their lives. Go out of your way to have uplifting experiences.

You may have to really want and choose to be well to start the healing process. This condition is biochemical, but our thoughts have a great impact on our outcomes. Be brave enough to turn it all around. There is no rule that says we cannot recover, at least in degrees. Even small steps help.

In about 600 BC, Taoist Lao Tzu said, 'A journey of a thousand miles begins with a single step.'

I encourage you to take that step.

Seven: Rebecca

I don't remember the first time I cut myself intentionally.

My family say I was always 'highly strung'. My father died when I was two years old and this is when my insomnia began. It has plagued me ever since. My mother was three months pregnant when he died, and my sister was born almost completely deaf. Before the age of five, she had a number of operations to correct her hearing, and during those times I was sent to my grandmother's house.

My grandmother and I never got along, and my memories of her during my childhood involve my being either hit or screamed at. I held a lot of resentment towards my mother for leaving me in my grandmother's care, and, to be honest, I still do. Aside from that, my childhood was fairly good.

At the tender age of eleven, I found an outlet for my frustration and a way to escape my emotional pain. A metal compass was the tool I used to injure myself during my first two years of high school, until someone caught on and took it away from me. By then I had moved on to bigger and better things, and I had also, for the most part, stopped cutting my arms and moved on to my legs so no one could see the damage I inflicted upon myself.

This was not my only act of secrecy. I hid razor blades behind the lining of my glasses case for 'emergencies' and perfected the art of removing the blade of my pencil sharpener, cutting, then putting it back before anyone noticed. I would buy a packet of cheap plastic pens each week, break them and use the sharp edges to scratch or cut myself. The pens and sharpener stayed in my pencil case as normal school items, although eventually one of my friends caught on to the sharpener and took that away too. I was quite inventive in ways to injure myself and avoid my scars or fresh cuts being exposed.

I became an excellent forger of my mother's handwriting and signature, which was very useful for informing the school about my imaginary skin condition. I would rather have died than be seen by my peers in bathers. My self-loathing, which led to self-harm, stemmed from my hatred of my own personality and body, and directly led to my inability to have normal relationships for many years.

I experienced my first serious bout of depression at age thirteen. The trigger was thought to be my friend Karen's diagnosis of terminal cancer. All these years later, there is still a faint scar on the back of my left hand from where I rubbed off the skin while our teacher told the class how sick Karen was. I rubbed the skin off with an eraser because, by that stage, my friends had rid my pencil case of anything sharp or anything I could possibly break and make sharp.

Karen's death affected me profoundly. I felt I should have been the one to die because I was worthless; I didn't deserve to live but Karen did. This idea was to stay with me for a decade. Despite the time that has passed, I still find it difficult to discuss Karen's death. My response to her death had a marked effect on those I was close to, both friends and family. I became angry with people I cared about because I was convinced they would leave me – either that, or I felt they were stupid for caring about someone who did not deserve to be cared about. I was certain I would die young and believed everybody would be happier without me in their lives.

I now have blank periods in my memory from that time, memories so painful that my mind has hidden them. There is a three-week time frame, from the moment I found out Karen was sick, that remains a complete mystery to me. I only remember the pain of watching her fade away, the pronounced increase in my own self-hatred, issues with trusting and caring for people, and constantly wishing I was the one who was sick and had died in her place.

I first attempted suicide at fifteen years of age. Now, aged 25, I've lost count of the number of times I have attempted to take my own life, but I estimate it to be around forty. The most eventful attempt involved a bottle of tequila, ingesting every pill I could get my hands on and trying to drive into a tree.

My psychiatrist and I had a discussion that went as follows:

Shrink: What happened?

Me: Clearly, I tried to kill myself.

Shrink: Then what happened?

Me: Well, obviously, I was unsuccessful. Otherwise I wouldn't be sitting here telling you this now, would I?

Shrink: Why were you unsuccessful?

Me: I told you! The drugs you put me on screwed up my depth-perception, so I missed the bloody tree!

Shrink: Then what happened?

Me: I went for the next tree!

Shrink: And what happened with that one?

Me: Umm, well, that one didn't actually exist …

By the age of sixteen, my mood swings had increased in severity and I began to experience manic and psychotic episodes. My doctor prescribed antidepressants. Unfortunately, I had a manic or psychotic episode nearly every time I started on them, and I was frustrated by the fact that this didn't seem to alert my doctors that something wasn't right! However, in their defence, I wasn't exactly honest with them. I didn't realise the 'highs' were bad. So I'd stop taking the antidepressants when I felt good (manic) without telling them, and go back the next time I crashed, saying that the previous drug didn't work.

I've been prescribed at least a dozen different tablets, but there are two that had side-effects of particular note. My experience with the first was truly horrible. I couldn't sleep and was constantly agitated, sweaty, anxious and zombie-like. Eventually I stopped taking it and ended up having a full-blown manic episode to mark the occasion.

The second drug was the most vile substance I have ever had the displeasure of encountering. My body certainly thought so, anyway. Within half an hour of taking my first dose, I was having horrible pains, coupled with the distinct feeling that an elephant was sitting on my chest. I couldn't breathe properly. I attempted to be sick but couldn't because my throat had closed up. I broke out in hives. I couldn't stop shaking. I had cold sweats. I felt dizzy. I had trouble with my vision and experienced 'black spots', horrific episodes during which a massive black spot would appear in my line of sight, overtake everything else, render me blind and then recede again. I honestly believed I was going to die.

All of the medication I tried (including the hideous drugs mentioned above) had the same effect. I'd feel better for a few weeks, and then I'd 'go nuts', stop taking them and end up attempting suicide or engaging in other irrational behaviour.

Of course everyone is different, so the medication that works for one may not work for another. It's a process of trial and error.

The worst injury I inflicted upon myself was at school, at age sixteen. I was heavily into 'The Manic Street Preachers' band at the time. One band member, Richie, carved the term '4REAL' into his arm during an interview when asked if the band was 'for real'. He cut down to the bone, as I recall. I remember being fed up with feeling 'numb' and people thinking that I was an 'attention seeker', so I took a leaf out of his book, stole a knife from the Year Twelve common room and engraved those same characters into my right thigh. I bled to unconsciousness.

Throughout this period of my life, I really did want to die. It's almost impossible to explain to someone who has never done it, but when I was upset like that and near hysterical, self-injury had the same effect on me as a Valium does on many others. I could feel the intense emotions under my skin and thought that I'd die from them. The more I bled the calmer I felt, until I was back in control.

Up until the age of nineteen, I was 'all over the place'. When I started smoking, I developed a fondness for putting lit matches on my breasts to inflict injury. Some people take drugs to escape reality; some people develop eating disorders to escape themselves. I don't see my self-injury as a means of escape. I see it as a way to cope and control my emotions and a way to bring me back to reality when I am numb.

Whether or not I'll ever be 'cured' of this addiction (and it is very much an addiction), I don't know. My psychiatrist asks me at every appointment, 'Are you still self-mutilating?' – a term that I detest. I either say *yes* but refuse to elaborate, or lie and say *no*.

At 25 years old I made it to 96 days self-injury-free before I crashed.

The urge is always there, no matter how much I suppress it. It lurks in the back of my brain and I crave the release, the pleasure of the endorphin rush and the chill of it afterwards. It's similar to how most people see sex or an orgasm. The difference with me is that I dislike sex but love self-injuring.

I guess my dislike of sex stems again from my own self-loathing. The odd thing is I use sex in the same way I use self-injury – as a means to feel better about myself. Yet it has the opposite effect. I always feel revolting and disgusted afterwards.

While I've been able to somewhat overcome my urges to self-injure now, I find it almost impossible to discuss my issues about men and sex. I tend to come across as flirty, so people assume I've slept with a lot of men, which is about as far from the truth as you can get. Perhaps it's because every significant male figure in my life has disappointed me in some way; perhaps it's because I hate the self-inflicted scars on my body and feel the need to hide them from everybody – I don't know. Of the people I have slept with, I've only enjoyed sex with one, but I still couldn't shake the feeling of disgust afterwards. No matter how much I enjoy sex at the time, my mood always drops afterwards for about a week.

My romantic relationships generally fall into one of two categories:

the men who have feelings for me and the men I have feelings for. The two rarely, if ever, cross over. When it comes to the ones who have feelings for me, I find myself almost always incapable of feeling anything but contempt towards them for being stupid enough to love someone as toxic as I am. I end up dominating them and screwing them around. The more they love me, the more I end up hating them and wanting to make them feel pain. The way I view it is that they deserve it for loving someone who is not worthy of being loved.

The ones I have feelings for tend to confirm my view of myself and increase my own self-loathing because they don't care back. And even if they do, I convince myself they don't. To put it mildly, I start acting like a complete psycho Antichrist towards them and generally mess up their lives as much as possible before they finally tell me to take my bullshit somewhere else.

And thus the cycle continues – usually with me going back to one who cares for me and screwing him around until I feel better about myself.

At the age of twenty my moods became a problem when I moved to the other side of the city, away from all my friends and everything I knew. I had lived in the same area since I was born, and I hated where I was now living. I was a nightmare to be around and isolated myself from all the new friends I made. In a fit of mania I hacked my hair off (it was long enough for me to sit on), scrubbed at my hands and body until they bled and made life hell for everybody who came near me.

When my niece was born, I marked the occasion by having a psychotic episode the day she was brought home from the hospital. My grandmother had come over, and I was struggling to deal with my younger sister having a child. Instead of leaving me alone to get over it, she decided to start screaming at me for not being supportive of my sister and telling me how evil I was (something I was pretty used to hearing by this stage). After several hours of this, I finally cracked when I walked past her to go into my room and continue drinking the bottle of tequila I had started that day, and she grabbed my wrist.

If there is one thing I cannot stand more than anything when I'm like that, it's being touched. The result of this was getting into a full-on physical fight with her, calling her every filthy name I could think of and hitting her back every time she belted me. My mother threatened to call the police to come and get me, my sister called my best friend who brought over antipsychotic medication, my grandmother dumped a bottle of holy water over me because she thought I was possessed, and I ended up sitting in the corner of the kitchen on the floor, bashing my head repeatedly against the wall. Not my finest hour.

This period of my life was also marked with increasing drug and alcohol abuse and a series of unsuccessful relationships. The drug abuse stopped when I ended up in hospital after having a heart attack and being diagnosed with a heart condition. At the time I told myself the two were completely unrelated, as I'd had blood pressure problems since the age of sixteen. In retrospect, I see that the drugs made the condition a lot worse than it would have been and may have even caused it. Because of them, I may need a pacemaker by the time I'm thirty.

What really bothers me is that the medications needed for my heart don't particularly like the medications I need for bipolar disorder. When I have trouble with one condition, the other condition is neglected and often worsens because of a need to change medication.

At 21 years old, my life took another twist. A man came into my life. He was a customer from work and became both my lover and closest friend, until I did something very unlike me. I fell in love.

This was something I was completely unable to deal with, and I made his life hell because of it. It should also be noted that there was a marked increase in my self-injuring during this time. I lost what little self-worth I had. I hated myself and even hated him, though I also loved him at the same time.

Irrational behaviour was my forté, so I thought at the time that I should try and hurt him as much as possible because he had hurt me by making me love him. Why that hurt me, I don't know, but it did. I tried a number of times to unsuccessfully cut him out of my life, which never worked. I also tried to not love him, which again didn't work.

And then he was diagnosed with cancer.

I don't think I've ever 'lost the plot' as badly as I did then. Everything that had haunted me since Karen's death came back. All the pain, hurt and anger from her illness and death seemed to blend into the pain, hurt and anger I felt towards this friend getting sick. Try as I might, I couldn't separate the two. I felt I had nowhere to turn and nobody to talk to about how I was feeling. So I turned my rage inwards and took it out on myself.

I was completely convinced the thoughts I'd formed and maintained since Karen's death were right. It was my fault my lover was sick because I loved him and everything I touched was poisoned by the darkness in me. I can't even begin to put into words the shame I now feel at the way I acted during his illness.

While he had chemotherapy, I went through one of the most severe depressive episodes I've ever endured. I had a massive fight with my friend, who told me I needed to do something about my moods, so I went to see a doctor. The amusing thing about this is that I agreed to see a doctor out of spite, to prove that it was he who had the problem, not me. But for once in my life, I was completely honest, telling the doctor about the highs as well as the lows. After some increasingly bizarre questions, he told me that he suspected I had bipolar disorder. I was referred to a psychiatrist, who confirmed the diagnosis.

My first reaction was intense relief. Despite how miserable I was feeling, I was glad that there was an explanation for what was wrong with me. I wasn't just 'crazy' – there was a medical reason behind my thoughts and behaviour.

I started on a drug that made me feel worse than I had ever felt before, and this period of my life was marked with a number of suicide attempts and psychotic episodes. It took over a year to find a drug combination that worked: a combination of mood stabilisers, antipsychotics and sedatives. During this time I was also diagnosed with chronic generalised anxiety disorder, panic disorder and agoraphobia.

The agoraphobia began when a new manager started at work. She was apparently convinced that I would blow up our workplace or start stabbing customers left, right and centre because I had bipolar. She made my life hell for a few months before the union got involved. I ended up having a complete breakdown. I couldn't leave the house, could barely get out of bed, couldn't look after myself and would go days without sleeping. I then experienced what was known as 'bipolar rage'. I pretty much just screamed and cried and abused everyone and everything that came near me. The only good thing that can be said about my breakdown was that I completely lacked the motivation to attempt to kill myself. I couldn't even get in the shower on my own, let alone organise a suicide.

I hated my medication with a passion. The thing that annoyed me most about it was the metallic taste I had in my mouth. I have no idea why it bothered me so much, but it drove me insane! When they increased my dose I could also smell it on my skin and in my hair, which made me slightly obsessive-compulsive. I'd shower eight or nine times a day and brush my teeth countless times. Other 'delights' included never being able to remain hydrated (it got so bad I had to drink Gastrolyte every day – this is normally used to treat dehydration from diarrhoea). I would sweat constantly. I had kidney problems and repeated urinary tract infections. My eyesight became poor and my skin looked like it was being eaten by bugs. There was also the issue of weight gain. On one occasion, they increased my dose and I gained nine kilos in ten days. That was the final straw, and I swapped medications.

Just before they switched my medications over, I had another psychotic episode, which was brought on from my constant stopping and starting this drug. I hurled abuse and death threats at my friend (the one I was in love with) for weeks. This ended with yet another suicide attempt and almost landed me in hospital.

Somewhere between threatening to kill him and attempting to kill myself, he called the intake centre at a local hospital that had a psychiatric ward. They phoned me and I went berserk, threatening to set fire to their cars and body parts if they came anywhere near me. I told them that I would drive myself off a bridge if I so much as felt they were going to admit me. They ended up calling my friend back and suggesting he call both an ambulance and the police to get me under control and admitted. Their mistake was calling me back and telling me this. I stormed out of the house and called my friend on my mobile to shriek more abuse at him, along with the most horrible insults I could think of. I spent that night sitting by the freeway, contemplating throwing myself under every truck that went past.

Two weeks later I decided I couldn't forgive him for the events of that night and told him to get out of my life, once again dragging up every filthy insult I could think of and getting a tattoo to mark the occasion, which says *lovers are lunatics – know thyself.* You can count the number of major episodes I've had by the number of tattoos I have. I didn't speak to him for nearly a year. I also took a year off sex and relationships, and isolated myself from everyone to try and work out some of my issues. It's the best thing I've ever done. Not only did I manage to get over my feelings for him, which in turn allowed me to be friends with him again, but I began to work with a psychologist to figure out a lot of my unresolved issues, some of which I didn't even know bothered me.

I also took time to work out what triggers my episodes and how to avoid those triggers or deal with them if they occurred. I was able to focus enough to turn my attention to starting the Australian Bipolar Schizoaffective Network.

Everyone is different, but to me, bipolar disorder is staying awake for days at a time, feeling your skin crawl and being unable to sit still for more than thirty seconds. It's wondering if the things you see out of the corners of your eyes are actually there or whether it's because you haven't slept for a week. It's being so low you don't have the energy to get out of bed, let alone have a shower or leave the house.

It's having static bounce around the inside of your skull until you are half mad with it. It's paranoia, anxiety, remorse; thinking and talking too fast to make any sense, and rage with those you love for no reason. It's drinking a bottle of vodka and taking handful after handful of whatever pills you can get just to stop the noise in your head and put an end to everything else you feel.

It's being unable to hold down a job. It's self-loathing. It's seeing a psychiatrist who probes into your head until you are admitting things you previously refused to admit to yourself. It's wondering how much your friends and family hate you after your last episode. It's wondering what damage you will do in your next episode.

It's completely screwing up your finances until you've got banks bashing down your door because you maxed out a credit card in a week during a manic episode, then couldn't pay it back. It's knowing that you'll never have financial security.

It's feeling and being treated like a child because you are incapable of looking after yourself or have no sense of danger. It's heaven, it's hell ... all this and so much more!

Over the last three years, I have worked with a psychologist and begun removing the seeds I planted in my mind as a child. He gives me the tools to figure things out for myself. Though it's hard, it's beneficial and satisfying. I'm much more positive now. I have gained an insight into what makes my mind work in the way it does, which benefits me a great deal.

I have chronic generalised anxiety and panic disorders with agoraphobia. My medication helps me function when I have anxiety and don't want to leave the house. It also helps my panic attacks, especially since someone suggested putting it under my tongue while I'm having an attack.

I've also gained a lot more self-worth. I now realise there are situations I can change and those I can't; that there is no point stressing over things I can't change, and that I make the choice to stress.

My interest in Buddhism has helped me immensely. Through reading books by the Dalai Lama, I've discovered how to forgive and how little things really don't matter in the long term.

In November 2006, I started the MySpace Aussie Bipolar group. The one thing that kept coming up in this group was the severe lack of support groups and the cost of those that were around. In December 2007 I started the Australian Bipolar Schizoaffective Support website and began running support groups through it. From there I began to turn it into a non-government non-profit organisation, and I hope to eventually turn it into the first Bipolar and Schizoaffective Foundation in Australia.

The aim of the Australian Bipolar Schizoaffective Support Network (ABSSN) is to provide a safe, free and supportive place for those who are diagnosed with bipolar or schizoaffective disorders. The network has expanded to include resources and support for those with a dual diagnosis or with anxiety disorders, and incorporates separate support for teens and carers, as well as providing resources for suicide prevention and self-injury support. I am also working to include postnatal depression and psychosis, and substance abuse support and resources.

My long-term aims, after turning ABSSN into a foundation, include establishing grants for those who struggle to pay for their medication and psychiatric treatment, and running awareness campaigns to make ABSSN known to those who would benefit from the services and support offered, as well as to the general public. I hope to begin eliminating the stigmas associated with bipolar, schizophrenia and schizoaffective disorders.

I intend to establish a recovery house for those who need a safe place to stay when their illness feels like it is too much to deal with on their own. They will have access to whatever medical treatment they need, paid for by ABSSN, if necessary, and will be around others who understand what they are going through. They will be given the opportunity to engage in a variety of activities that can be used as coping techniques.

Through establishing ABSSN, I realised how much being able to talk to other people who were in my situation and feeling the same things I was, helped me deal with my own diagnosis. I've come into contact with some of the most amazing people I will ever meet and I will be eternally grateful to those who have helped me along my journey. People involved with ABSSN have brought positive energy into my life. I'm also eternally grateful to those who have been there, not only through my journey with bipolar, but through everything else.

I have bipolar disorder, but it does not have me. So many people I speak to refer to themselves 'as' bipolar. I don't. I refer to myself by my name and if it happens to come up in conversation, then yes, I do have bipolar disorder. It does not control me, I control it (most of the time anyway!). I don't lose my sense of self to it. All that I am, and all that I will be, is not merely a mental illness. I am so much more than that. And yet, you may wonder, how can I say that, when one of my goals in life is to raise as much awareness of bipolar as possible? How can I say that, when I am currently working to build a non-profit organisation for it and spend most of my time working on my bipolar website?

Easily. I do it so I am the one in control. I do it so others out there can gain some control too. I do it so people who fear and stereotype those with bipolar disorder will one day see that we are not just labels – 'bipolar', 'crazy', 'dangerous', 'psycho', 'nuts' – or any of the other stigmas attached to severe mental illness. We are all individuals with different thoughts, feelings, emotions, memories, likes, dislikes, loves, opinions, passions and talents like all the other people in the world.

These days I'm very close to my sister and niece. My sister is one of my closest friends and is a constant source of inspiration to me. My niece is now five years old and the one person in the world who can make me smile at absolutely any time. Her innocence and love for me touch me in a way nothing else can. When she had chicken pox earlier this year, the only thing that made her feel better was sleeping in my bed (even though it meant I got no sleep!). I love taking her out for coffee – I have my short black and she feels very grown up with her babychino. I've been playing tuned percussion since I was nine years old; then I learnt to play drums and percussion, and later, viola. Now I'm learning the flute! I love music and plan to teach my niece how to play either the viola or violin soon.

I read extensively. I also write stories and poetry. Poetry is a wonderful release for me and really helps express what I'm feeling.

When I began to research my family history, I realised my bipolar is a genetic thing. Several of my relatives had mental illness and some were simply 'not all there'!

I enjoy spending way too much money on red lipstick and T.U.K. platform heels. I love working in the garden and have a particular passion for bonsai. I adore travelling. I have visited thirteen countries so far. I'm interested in Greek and Roman mythology and one of my (many) tattoos is part of an inscription on the Temple of Apollo in Delphi.

I truly believe that one person can make a difference, and that no matter how hard or high the mountain is to climb, it can be done – and with style! And that, regardless of our diagnosis, we are limited only by our own imaginations. We can achieve the amazing, the seemingly impossible, and whatever our hearts desire.

Eight: Imogen

Some people experience mental illness only once and fully recover. For others, it continues throughout their lives. I am one of the latter.

At the age of eighteen I was accepted into university so I moved out of home and into a boarding college. I was beginning to experience quite lengthy and severe mood swings at this stage of my life, though nothing like the full-blown mania I would later experience. Throughout my university years I slid from having drive and energy into the isolation and hopelessness of depression.

After completing my degree, I was accepted into the honours program in anthropology. I turned this down in order to relocate interstate. Such a dramatic change in circumstances was very stressful and difficult at first, but I felt strongly that it was what I needed to do with my life. After a number of changes in living arrangements, I moved into shared accommodation with a flatmate.

In the midst of this I also travelled to New Zealand. My boyfriend of the time was a university lecturer working in Christchurch, so I went to visit him for the last three months of his employment. It was after this visit, upon our return to Australia, that the first severe signs of illness became apparent.

I returned home to my family for Christmas for the first time in three years and entered into a stage of full-blown mania. I started to experience euphoric moods, surges of ideas, impatience, fast speech, a decreased need for sleep and a distracted mind. Despite my parents' concern, I decided to return to home after the festivities, and travelled back interstate.

I was acting so strangely that the friend I returned with wanted nothing more to do with me after that trip. My flatmate had no idea what to do with me either. I paced the floor and talked at a hundred miles an hour. Someone (it may have even been me) rang my boyfriend. In the end my boyfriend's brother (who was a surgeon) came over, took one look at me and said, 'She's manic. We need to get her to hospital!'

Next, I recall being at the hospital and talking to the psychiatrist. I rambled irrationally to him and was given a very strong injection. I woke up next morning in the psychiatric ward and stayed there for three months. It was during this hospitalisation in 1995 that I was diagnosed with bipolar disorder at the age of 23 years.

I was completely psychotic at the time, and high as a kite. I began to believe that I was Anastasia, the Russian tsar's long-lost daughter. I then became convinced that I had attended the National Institute of Dramatic Arts (NIDA) and that I was, in fact, a famous actress. I later believed that I was Olivia Newton-John (even in my later hospitalisations I would borrow the video of the musical *Grease* and perform the role of Sandy). Sometimes I would associate with what I read in magazines and believe the experiences I read about were my own. This was particularly so when reading about Olivia Newton-John following her breast cancer surgery. I also believed that everyone I met was related to me because we were all descendants of Father Abraham. I used unusual (and often amusing) names to identify close family and friends.

Many of the other patients were struggling with extreme issues, including anorexia. Witnessing their struggles was a real challenge but it gave me a much broader perspective on life. It was a real eye-opener. I also saw people released from care who didn't seem well at all.

I actually enjoyed that hospital stay because I was euphoric at the time. I don't recall the irritability that has been a symptom of my later episodes of mania. I had a heightened sense of *joie de vivre*, though I was also prone to confusion. Even now my memories of this time are very one-sided and hazy.

I experienced my most severe delusions during this period, but I have had visual and/or auditory hallucinations at other times. Once I lived on the top floor of a two-storey apartment building. On one occasion, I heard a group of kids outside throwing rocks on the roof. I went to speak with my neighbour about it, and he pointed out that there were no kids outside and he couldn't hear anything hitting the roof. On another occasion I heard someone trying to climb through the manhole in my ceiling, to get into my apartment. It was frightening. I later realised that my apartment didn't have a manhole.

After leaving hospital I completed my studies and moved back to live with my parents. My boyfriend was against the move so I lost his support and we broke up. I spent a lot of time with the animals and did arts and crafts, which helped to keep me calm. It was actually very good therapy for me.

I found a new psychiatrist and things started going really well. To my absolute delight, I was offered a twelve-month contract to teach English to students in Japan. At the time, it felt like a dream come true. I was assigned to a country town in Japan where very little English was spoken. I taught evening classes while most of the other English teachers taught during the daytime; this made socialising very difficult. It wasn't what I expected at all. I found the life very hard and was extremely lonely. Toward the end I got drunk and tried to overdose on Lithium to forget things. Eventually I was hospitalised with depression.

The language barrier in hospital was a real problem. None of the nurses spoke English and the psychiatrist didn't speak enough English for me to stay on in Japan under his care. In the end my mother came all the way to Japan to collect me. Teaching English overseas had been a deep ambition of mine since completing my degree, and now it was falling apart at the seams. Having had to quit my twelve-month contract after only three months, I believed I had failed.

After I left the hospital, my mother and I spent several days in a Japanese hotel waiting for a flight back to Australia. I felt trapped by my feelings and was desperate to run away from everything. I continued to feel very depressed and by this stage I was suicidal. I would get up in the middle of each night and try to sneak out of the hotel, so neither my mother nor I got much sleep. I was bitterly angry at what I saw as my absolute failure and took it out on my mother. She tried to distract me, but I was so despondent that nothing worked. Everything reminded me of my perceived failure.

When it came time to leave Japan, the airline staff were very helpful. They cleared an entire row of seats so I could lie down and gave me a blanket to increase my comfort. I kept trying to figure out a way to open the aircraft doors and jump out.

When we arrived back in Australia, I was admitted to a psychiatric hospital again for a lengthy period. I didn't want anyone to know I was in hospital and it wasn't until I was discharged that anyone besides my immediate family knew I had even returned from Japan. I was in a severe state of depression at the time, and believed I was in a women's prison rather than a hospital – and given the routines and practices, anyone could be forgiven for believing so. When deeply depressed I would find it hard to get up in the mornings; however, hospital routine dictated that if a patient wasn't on time for breakfast, they missed out. Patients were not allowed to eat breakfast any later than the scheduled time.

Although I believed most of the nursing staff of this particular institution treated me with rudeness and hostility, there was one intern who tried very hard to engage me. However, I had completely shut myself off and I wouldn't talk to anyone, so the doctor set up additional appointments for me with a psychologist. I found this to be a complete waste of time. The psychologist would talk for so long that the intern assumed progress was being made. But this wasn't the case, so a meeting was arranged for me with the head psychiatrist; but I wouldn't talk to him either. After our short meeting, he incorrectly diagnosed me as suffering from schizoaffective disorder. I had already been diagnosed with bipolar affective disorder type 1 and, apart from this incident, my diagnosis has never changed.

I continued to experience guilt about leaving Japan and believed I had failed at the only thing I had wanted to do with my life, which was to travel the world by teaching overseas.

During this time, I was eventually able to engage with one person, a woman from the pastoral care team who sometimes came in to visit patients. Somehow I managed to talk with her. However, nothing really changed and eventually I returned home still depressed.

I believed I had no future, but once I arrived home I slowly started to recover. I continued to see my mental health team and was referred to a local community health nurse whose patience and care were immeasurable. Over time, I reconsidered what the future had in store. I decided to work with kindergarten children so I took a volunteer role. This fulfilling work, along with the support of my out-patient mental health team, helped to pull me out of my low state and my future began to look brighter.

I enrolled in a Graduate Bachelor of Early Childhood Education at university and moved house, ready to commence a year of full-time study. Things went really well at first: I felt completely recovered. If times got tough, I found the Rural & Remote Mental Health Service team very helpful. However, by second semester I was falling apart. I still found travelling to university exhausting, and I had to repeat the field placement as well as keep up with all the other assignments that were due.

Luckily I recognised my early warning signs: not eating or sleeping well; rapid speech; fast flowing ideas; inappropriate elation; promiscuous behaviour. One morning, after staying up partying the entire night before without any sign of tiredness, I recognised that I was experiencing another high. I was determined not to return to the previous psychiatric hospital so I went to my local hospital. By the time I was admitted I was extremely manic. I spent months in the psychiatric unit of this hospital.

During this hospital stay, very strong medication was used to bring me down and it had terrible side-effects. I had strong muscle spasms and would shuffle around with my head attached to my shoulder. What a look!

However, many positive changes started happening in my life after that hospital stay. I transferred my studies from early childhood to adult education. I moved into a two-bedroom flat and started studying at a different university. I was assigned a new mental health nurse whose support was invaluable.

My psychiatrist told me of a wonderful organisation known as the Mood Disorders Association (MDA). MDA had a support group where young people met to share their experiences, and I encountered enormous support within this group. I was able to go along and talk openly. I discovered that there were other people in similar circumstances and, most importantly, no one judged me. I began to realise that I had limitations and that it was vital to remain on my medication, so periods of wellbeing and stability started to extend substantially. Hospitalisation is now a rare occurrence.

I can't emphasise enough how important community care has been for me. Although hospital admission is vitally important when I am acutely sick, I have found that the environment escalates my mania because it's overstimulating; these days I'm better off at home with the support of a mental health team.

Developing a mental illness has resulted in many losses for me, including careers, relationships, study plans and financial security. I have experienced both depression and mania, and now realise that every high will be followed by a low and that the depth of this low depends on the height of the high. I cope well with my condition most of the time, but when I do recognise the signs of becoming unwell, I take responsibility and go to hospital seeking help. What frustrates me is the fact that when this happens, I am often confronted with rude and frustrated medical practitioners who ask what I think

I'm doing there. 'You look well to me,' they say, and send me home.

Yes, I look well, and I usually manage my condition very well. But I know when I need help. They don't see the dark side. They don't see how many times I have engaged in reckless risk-taking behaviour. They don't understand the times I have desperately wanted to die. They don't seem to recognise what's going on underneath. Sometimes I am simply not believed when I explain how I am feeling. They weigh it up: usually I'm well; I'm able to live independently and I study and/or have a job. They spare no more than about twenty minutes and don't hear anything I say before abruptly sending me home.

I'm able to manage now much of the time without needing hospitalisation because I have an exceptional private psychiatrist who knows me well and treats me with respect. I have been working with this psychiatrist for several years and I am able to get in contact at any time.

My delusions and hallucinations have continued to diminish over time and recede with each subsequent hospitalisation. To begin with, they were strong and persistent, but now I rarely get any at all. I still get highs and lows and occasionally experience panic attacks, but in general I am very well. I attribute much of my recovery to having had the same excellent psychiatrist for a long period of time, to receiving medications that suit me, and to having a supportive husband and family. I have been married for four years. Although my husband also has a mental illness, we are able to support each other and have a rich, happy and fulfilling life.

I have found that educating myself about my condition has been extremely helpful. I continue to attend forums, discussions and lectures, and read self-help literature about other people's experiences of living with bipolar disorder. I used to be passionate about breaking down stigmas in society, and as a member of the Mental Illness Fellowships education group I often spoke to members of the community about the signs and symptoms of bipolar disorder and my own experience.

Unfortunately, there are still some members of society who view people with a mental illness as 'nutcases', 'loonies' or 'psychos'. The media in particular tend to portray people with a mental illness as dangerous and violent rather than, more accurately, as confused and frightened.

When I was a community educator I was completely open with people about my illness. But now, unless I specifically want to educate someone about bipolar disorder, I don't mention it. I currently work as a home tutor, having worked in a wide variety of jobs. I find that work can sometimes be draining and stressful but it is also vital to my wellbeing, as I need to keep busy and be around others. I have never really stuck at any job for long, usually because a manic episode interferes, but I like to try different things and I know when it's time to move on.

I share the same hopes and dreams as anyone else. My greatest challenge is not being able to have children. I would find it too stressful to manage. As hard as it is, the truth is that I have limits and can't do everything. I've come to realise that to be healthy, I need to put my health before everything else. Some people don't understand this but honestly, it is the key to my wellness.

I have a list of strategies that help me, particularly when I am manic. I find classical music very soothing, as well as relaxation tapes and aromatherapy. I also find that being physically active is good for my health. I enjoy walking, especially bushwalking, and riding my bike. We have a dog, a very lively beagle, whom I love taking for walks along the creek near our house. I'm also addicted to crosswords. Some people don't understand how I could possibly find crosswords relaxing, but I do. They help me 'switch off' from everything else.

I avoid coffee and don't do anything over-stimulating. Keeping busy at home is important too, and I enjoy both photography and making gift cards for friends and family. I am involved with an arts group for people with a disability. My husband and I love to travel. We have visited Vietnam, Thailand, Dubai, Malta and Sicily.

Being with immediate family brings me great pleasure. I am lucky enough to have two adorable nieces and a nephew.

Overall I am both happy and healthy these days but I appreciate the fact that I have been blessed with a caring support network.

One of the most important things I have learned is that there is nothing more potent than a powerful outlook! If you live with a mental illness, I encourage you to keep believing in yourself, your hopes and your dreams, and don't let anyone's misconceptions stand in your way.

Nine: Michael

I grew up all around Australia because my dad was in the army. I saw 90 per cent of Australia by the time I was seventeen years old and then experienced the rest when I too joined the army. I enjoyed travelling around and I still do.

I was the younger of two brothers. My brother was a pain in the arse but older brothers usually are. We used to hate each other's guts, get into fist fights and beat each other black and blue. There was no love lost between us.

I didn't have any symptoms of mental illness when I was a kid. I was pretty steady all the way through, really. There is no history of similar illness in my family except for my Dad, and his problems came from Vietnam. Nothing wrong from my grandparents, they were OK. It was just part of my life back then – it was always pretty hard.

The more I stayed away from home the happier I was. I used to do bad things but I used to have a ball. I didn't have any anger issues when I was a kid except towards my brother. But that's only because of what he did to me. I got my own back eventually and it stopped happening after I punched him out a few times.

My parents tried to tar me with their brush but it didn't work. If my old man said *run* I'd walk. If he said *black* I'd say white. I used to get the blame for everything that happened when my brother and I were growing up around the house.

He used to say, 'He did it. He did it,' and I'd say, 'You lying bastard.' Next thing I'd get a smack around the ear from Dad, saying, 'Don't you lie.'

'Oh yeah, righto Dad.' Then I would pull my brother aside, hang onto him and say, 'Stick it up your arse.'

It got into a cycle. My brother would go and tell Dad that I had done something, so I'd go and give him a flogging and say, 'If you try it again I'll come and give you another one.'

My dad would come along and ask what happened. My brother would say, 'Well, he did it,' and I'd say, 'Yep, righto.' My father would give me a flogging so I'd go and give my brother another flogging. I'd say, 'Don't you dare tell Pa what happened.'

When I was growing up, it wasn't bad but it wasn't good either. I learned to just be myself more than anything else. Because of the things I went through, the things I had to go through, it's made me a better person today.

When I was at school people thought I was a bully but I wasn't. I used to go and beat up on the kids who would beat up all the lesser kids. If they were the same size I'd say, fight your own battles, but if someone wasn't as strong I'd stand up for them. I used to stick up for all the non-conformists and the different types. I was a rebel when I was growing up – no two ways about it.

At about ten years old, I was lighting fires – grass fires. I always had a firebug in me and I still have, but my later stint in the army taught me to control my outward aggression.

That same year I had my first incident with the coppers. I was in Melbourne at the time and decided to go shoplifting in Myer's. There was me, my mate and my brother. We had big parkas on and we were filling our pockets up. It was about our seventh time when we got caught. They took us to the cop shop, which was attached to the shopping centre. I was just sitting there but my brother was bawling his eyes out. 'You're a bloody wimp!' I told him.

He said, 'Dad's going to kill me.'

I said, 'I don't give a shit what Dad does to you. I'm going to get a flogging and I don't care.'

There were also two girls there. They were perhaps two or three years older than us and they had been caught stealing dresses. Each one had about seven dresses on underneath their own dress. They were bawling their eyes out as well, and I said, 'Don't worry about it, girls, you'll be all right. It's just a part of life.'

When the coppers called my parents they decided to leave us down there to stew for a while. It didn't bother me. We had been caught at about eleven o'clock in the morning and Mum and Dad didn't come until about five o'clock in the afternoon. They walked in to see me sitting there with a big smirk on my face.

Dad said, 'You know I'm going to wipe that smirk off your face when we get home?'

I said, 'Yeah, I know you will.'

We got home and sure enough, smack, smack, smack. My brother didn't get a finger laid on him but I did. My brother just blamed me. It went on from there.

Another time, I was told by police to empty my pockets. In them, I had about four padlocks with safety pins made out as keys. The copper said, 'Oh, you're stealing mail from mailboxes too. That's a federal offence.'

I said, 'Nuh, these padlocks are mine. I just lost the keys.'

'Why have you got four of them, then?'

'I collect padlocks. What's wrong with that?'

He didn't believe me.

I never stole mail. I used to blow up mail boxes. I did it for the hell of it – because I could. I think the main reason was that my parents tried to mould me to a way they wanted and I refused. I didn't want to be like them.

I think that most of the things I did were a sort of protest against what my parents would do to me. They'd say, 'You're a good boy, Michael,' and I'd say, 'Like hell I am.' I'd go and do things to spite them. Admittedly I was lucky and didn't get caught for most of the things I did – if I had it would probably be a different story – but I was very lucky. Someone was watching over me.

Mum was a hypochondriac because of the old man. The old man was never there so I was the one who sort of looked after her. She used to ask why I'd disappear for days at a time and I said it was because I could. I was out the door and gone.

Whenever she got hold of me she'd tell me to get inside and do my chores and I'd say, 'Yeah, OK, no worries.' I always did what she wanted eventually. It's hard to describe my mother really. She always came across more as the dutiful wife than the dutiful mother. She was always cooking, cleaning and ironing. I suppose that's what women were expected to do back in those days. Their focus was the man of the house more than the kids – the kids always took second place. And that basically was what happened in my house – I was less important.

But not my brother. He always got what he wanted. I never did. If I ever needed anything or got anything new, he would just go ahead and break it. I always used to get the blame for breaking my own things, but it was never me. Whenever I got anything, I used to treasure it and sort of never let it go because I never knew if I was going to get something like it ever again. That happened right throughout my life for as long as I can remember. That's the way it's always been.

I didn't have any friends at all during school. I knew a lot of people and I had the respect of a lot of people but I have never had any friends. No friends whatsoever. That's because of the old man and later because of the army life.

I didn't really have a good relationship with my mother. I'm not close to either of my parents. They couldn't tell you what I like or what I dislike, even to this day. The only reason I associate with my parents at all is because my father has a bike, and that's it. No other reason. If I were to walk past them in the street I wouldn't even stop to say g'day. Even if I knew my father just as a friend, there's no way in the world I'd go near him. 'No, sorry, I can't come over. Busy.' That's just the way things are.

I can understand my father, to a point. He was always pretty good to me before he went away to Vietnam, and it's only now, after I've been diagnosed with depression, that I can see that this was my old man's problem too. Having fought in Vietnam and seen the things he saw, he came back a completely changed man. I'll guarantee that everyone who went over to Vietnam came back completely changed. They were hard-arsed bastards when they came back because of what happened over there, the way they had to face death. One minute you're there and the next minute you aren't.

Probably the biggest incident was when my brother tried out for Duntroon. The day before he left, we got into an argument and I beat the crap out of him. I broke his nose, fractured a cheekbone, gave him two black eyes and injured his shoulder so badly he couldn't lift his arm. When he got back, he said, 'I didn't get into Duntroon because of you.' I said it was because he was an arsehole that he didn't get in. He went and told the old man who came and gave me a flogging, so I gave my brother another one afterwards. I re-broke his nose, re-fractured his cheekbone and said, 'Don't do it again!' It was 1976 and I was fourteen.

My dad had no counselling before he went and no counselling when he got back. Even today, a lot of the people who went to the Gulf War are treated in the same way – 'Thanks for coming, see you later. You don't need help – piss off. I don't know you.'

Nowadays they have started to realise you *do* need help, and I say, give it to them. They need it. The problems can fester for many, many years afterwards and that was the case with my father.

My mother always took a background position in my life growing up. Dad was always boozing, pissed; and every time he'd come home Mum would say, 'Oi! Don't annoy your father,' so we all had to take a back seat. I know dad used to slap her around. So I confronted him one day when we were living in New Guinea. I was fifteen at the time. I saw two big holes in the laundry wall so I asked Mum, 'Where did they come from?'

'Oh, I just fell into the wall,' she said.

I said, 'No, Dad hit you, didn't he?'

She said, 'Don't you dare say anything!'

I said, 'Too bad!'

So I went up and asked him, 'What do you think you're doing hitting my mother?'

He just turned around and slam, knocked me down.

I said, 'If you ever do that again, I'm out of here. You'll never see me again.'

And he never repeated it because he knew he'd never see me again. After he hit me that time, I disappeared for a week. I was never more than 200 metres from home but they didn't know that. None of the other parents saw me, but I was just over at other kids' places. It put a scare into him because he never did it again.

I didn't really have any anger towards Mum. Not really. I know that there was nothing she could have done. If she had got up and said anything in my defence, he would have just slapped her back down. I hated my father for doing that.

He reckons he's never hit her but there have been too many bruises over the years for it to have been anything else. That's why I tried to stay away as much as I could because if I stayed home, I'd get a flogging. I'd just go out and about.

Living in New Guinea was great. I was fourteen, fifteen, sixteen when I was up there. The old man was always away somewhere drinking booze and I was always around other kids' places. They didn't have TV up there then but they did have movies. I'd go and watch movies every night of the week in New Guinea. I'd spend Friday and Saturday nights at the sailors' mess, Wednesday and Sunday nights at the car club, Monday nights at the yacht club, Tuesday nights at the officers' mess. I was never home. I was always out watching movies.

Or mucking around with other kids.

When you travel a lot you learn to keep to yourself because as soon as you make friends, you have to leave them. You are never in one place for long, so what's the point of making friends? You'd just be constantly disappointed and the heartache is just too much to handle when you're growing up. Friendships that are here one day and gone the next weren't for me.

Later, when I joined the army, I met a guy who came up and said, 'You're Michael, right?' and I said 'Yeah.'

'Don't you remember me?'

'Nuh.'

He told me his name was Paul someone-or-other and I thought, 'So?' Apparently we used to play football together in Cairns. He recognised me but I didn't recognise him. I suppose in a way I just didn't want to remember anyone.

They said the army would wipe me clean. I did enjoy my time in the army but I didn't really want to join. I didn't have a choice. I was working for a demolition yard in Melbourne at the time and I really loved that job. I loved destroying things.

I joined the army in 1979 at the age of seventeen. There was an MP standing next to me making sure that I signed.

When the old man took me to the recruiting centre on my first day, there were about thirty young kids sitting outside. My dad just walked straight up to the counter with me in tow and the guy behind the counter said, 'Come on straight through.' All those guys waiting just couldn't believe it.

The funny thing was that they didn't really give me a medical. When I saw the psych officer, he asked me a lot of questions such as, 'What do you think of homosexuality?'

I said, 'Oh, they're OK. I don't mind as long as they don't put their way on me.'

He said, 'What do you mean?'

I said, 'They have a right to live, don't they?'

Well, I knew that was not the answer the army was looking for in the 1970s. I was not suited to the army.

'Are you a racist?'

I said, 'Yep. I hate them with a bloody vengeance.'

Definitely not suited for the army.

The recruiting officer had the final say. He outweighed what the psych officer said. He sat down, looked at me and said, 'You don't remember me, do you Michael?'

Shit, I thought, I know the face. I said, 'I know your face.'

He said, 'Tassie.'

'Ah, Mr N.' He had been our next-door neighbour.

'The psych officer says you're not suited but I have the final say. You're in!'

I said, 'Yeah, thanks, good on you.' I didn't want to join and had said everything I could to screw it up but I just didn't have a choice. I was in whether I wanted to be or not. I became a signals communicator.

I spent fifteen years in the army. I'm glad now that I joined because it did put me on the straight and narrow. I also met my wife.

We first met just after I turned eighteen. We discovered we'd had the same circle of acquaintances for two years before we met. Meeting her was the best thing that ever happened to me. She saved my life. We got married in 1983; I was 21. We had our daughter when I was 25.

My wife and I spent about five years in Brisbane, and during that time we got married. Then we moved to Melbourne for two years, then back up to Brisbane for five years and over to Toowoomba for four years.

My illness was triggered in the army. I can't pin down a single cause – it was a combination of a lot of little things. The first one was the way I was treated medically. I broke my leg in 1982 playing football in the army, and I've had trouble with it ever since. The doctors really stuffed up the treatment.

There was one person in the army, the Regimental Sergeant Major, who thought I had broken my leg in a motorcycle accident and he hated motorcycles. He was in every unit I was in. The RSM held a lot of weight in those days. They sort of passed information down along the chain. If they thought you were a rabble-rouser or not worth anything you would get nothing.

He went to the Vietnam memorial in Canberra on one occasion and my parents were there too. My mum walked up to him and asked, 'How's my son going?'

He said, 'Oh, that bludging bastard?'

My old man said, 'What do you mean, bludging bastard?'

'He broke his leg in a motorcycle accident so he thinks he can get things on a silver platter.'

My father turned around and told him straight. 'Now you listen here, you dickhead, he didn't break his leg on a motorcycle. He broke his leg playing football. Go look at his medical documents and get your facts straight.'

Then there was the appalling way the army treated anyone they classed as an invalid. When you're sick or injured you can't get promoted because you've got to be fully fit to qualify for anything. As a soldier, you are in a catch-22 situation.

I was having a lot of trouble right up until around late 1985. I was pretty lucky actually that one of the female corporals said to me, 'Michael, if you want to learn to be a soldier you've got to stop being a layabout.'

I said, 'I'm not a layabout.'

She said, 'Yes you are.'

'I actually have a medical certificate,' I told her.

'You've got to learn to live with that and just get on with it. If you keep going the way you're going, they're going to discharge you,' she said.

That's when it clicked. I started to pull my finger out and pushed the injury aside as best I could. It made me a better person. Finally I started to get promotion courses in the army.

At the time I wasn't getting promotion courses or any more career progression courses. I wasn't even looking like getting them. It's really funny because after the RSM came back from Canberra, he signed me up for a Sergeant course. I wasn't getting panelled for it, I was getting straight in. The instructors in the course were told at the outset to leave me alone and I was the only one who wasn't picked on in the entire course. I passed the course.

I had been back two weeks and I was selected for platoon sergeant. Same thing again. I wasn't subject to panel selection and someone was removed from the course so that I could take his place. I wasn't harassed for the entire course.

I didn't find out why the army had changed their attitude until after I finished the courses and the old man told me what he had said. That really gave me a turn for the worse with my depression. When I found that out that everything that had happened to me in my military career was because of the RSM, I thought, 'You fucking arseholes.' It was because of him. That was the straw that broke the camel's back. It really sent me over the edge. 'Fuck the army!' I thought. 'They can go to hell!'

Here I was, I'd spent ten years in the army and I was only just being promoted. And there were all these other guys who had only been here two or three years and they were staff sergeants and warrant officers. It's pretty hard. I was basically an old soldier at 28, and I had warrant officers who were the same age or younger, giving me orders. I felt like telling them to go to hell because they were idiots. They had no idea what they were talking about. They hadn't been the time and rank that I had been. I had been a digger for ten years and it had made me a better person.

As I got older, I thought that if I ever got there I was going to look after my diggers. And I did. That's the difference between an old soldier and one who goes speeding through the ranks.

It makes a big difference and it also takes its toll. I don't care what anyone says – it does. It takes its toll. You have to listen to these young idiots who have no idea what they're talking about but you still have to call them *sir*. But as the old saying goes – you respect the rank, not the person.

All this pressure got on top of me and built up and built up and built up. I think that another contributing factor was how long I was away from home. Out of that particular four-year posting, I was away from home for about three-and-a-half years.

I started to notice a downhill slide with my depression and bipolar disorder around 1989 or 1990. That was when things were really starting to go bad, but at the time I just thought it was a normal part of life. I thought it was part of what the army does to you.

Back in those days I was hardly ever at home. I was always out bush so it made it hard, but it's also just the way the army trains you. Since I've been out of the army I've talked to a lot of guys who came out after twenty years. I tell them that I have bipolar disorder and they aren't surprised. Many of them have mates that developed bipolar disorder because of the army. That's what the army does to you. Right from the start the army trains you to the way they want you to think. If you think outside that square, you're toast. You haven't got a hope in hell so you end up conforming to their ways or you're shat on from a great height. You get nowhere. You get all the shit jobs under the sun, and I suppose that's the way it has to be.

When going out bush, you're supposed to have a three-man deck but we were going out in two-man detachments, which is really wrong because you get no sleep. One day out bush, I said, 'My boys are copping some sleep!' I said, 'You give my team an extra man,' and they cracked the shits at that.

That was the last bush trip I experienced before I flipped out and was checked into a mental health clinic. I wrote a sign saying *This is a bear-free zone so fuck off,* and I stuck it on my Rover. A major came up to me and said, 'I think that sign's rather inappropriate.'

I said, 'Fuck off!'

He said, 'I'll have you charged,' and that's when I leapt out of the back of the ute and landed on top of him. I grabbed him and said, 'You fuck off and leave my boys alone. I'm not doing your shit any more. Your boys bloody come back from time out in the bush. They have three square meals for the day. They get their clothes cleaned. They have a nice relaxing time during the day while we're out here picking up all this shit. Piss off, Sir, otherwise I'm packing up my vehicle and I'm out of here!'

He said, 'You'll be stopped at the first MP check point.'

I said, 'No, I fucking won't. They won't catch me!'

He said, 'I'll have you charged.'

I said, 'You do that Sir,' and then I whispered to him, 'I know where your kids go to school so you be careful what you do.'

It must have come across as though I really meant it, but really, I wouldn't have done anything to his kids. But he shat himself.

When we got back to the unit nothing was said at first. I told them that I had to get out of there before I killed someone. They told me that I had to see the psych officer but I refused as I didn't want it on my record. They assured me that it wouldn't go on my record. What a load of crap. Everything goes on your record. But I agreed to see him.

I told the psych officer not to give me a rifle again or I would shoot people. He asked who I would shoot. I told him at first that it was none of his business but then told him I'd start with a CO, three majors, three lieutenants and a sergeant. I told him I was deadly serious.

Then the Major said, 'Michael, come and talk to me.'

This was the first time they called me by my name. They usually referred to people by rank.

I said 'OK, no worries.'

The Major told me that I had to go to the hospital, so I went and they sent me on to the mental health clinic. Now the clinic I went to is probably very good, if you aren't in the military. But if you are in the military, it doesn't work. Their treatment programs are for civilians.

After this first time in the clinic, I was released and went back to the unit. I had to do what was known as a battle fitness test. This entailed an obstacle course, a carry test, then a sixteen-kilometre hike in two hours. I got over the obstacle course and decided not to continue. I thought it was a load of crap. My supervisor threatened to charge me and I told him to talk to my psych officer first. After that he left me alone. As soon as you mention the psych officer, they drop you like a hot spud because they can't mess with you. Having a psych officer is almost like confession in a church, it's sanctity. They can't touch it. After that day I didn't do Physical Training again.

Two weeks later I had to see the psychiatrist. The psychiatrists are military so they work for the government basically. They don't really do things the right way. He said he was going to put me back on full duties and I told him he was a fucking idiot. I got into my car and started driving back to Toowoomba. I didn't want to live.

I was speeding along and it was pissing down rain. I took the Murphy's Creek turn-off and decided that it was time to die. I took my hands off the steering wheel, put my foot flat on the accelerator and rolled the car.

The doctor at the hospital told me that the only thing that saved my life was that I relaxed. My shoulder was injured but that was all. The next day I was admitted back to the mental health clinic. And that's when the army decided they no longer wanted to know me.

I had been driving a military vehicle, so emergency services contacted the army and they sent someone from my unit out to see me. Usually the duty officer is sent, but for some unknown reason they sent out one of my own trade. So I knew straight away something was wrong.

The doctor, Major and the Matron put the paperwork in to get me discharged. My doctor was a fantastic bloke. I asked, 'So when am I going back?'

The doctor said, 'No, you're not going back. You're being discharged. The paperwork has already gone through,'

I didn't question it. I could have, I suppose, but I just didn't. I wasn't in any frame of mind, I didn't know if I was Arthur or Martha at the time.

There were only a handful of people in my unit who knew where I was. No one was told anything. Some of the guys from the unit asked my wife, 'Where's Michael?' and she'd say, 'I can't tell you that.' I told her to keep her mouth shut. I didn't want people to know where I was. It was none of their business.

The army wouldn't get me any clothes, they weren't bringing my wife down to see me, they weren't doing anything. Then my wife got a hold of the padre. The padre told the army to get me some clothes and arrange transport for my wife to see me. As soon as the padre got involved, boom! Things started moving, because you don't mess with padres or with psych officers.

On one of the trips back from seeing me, my wife was escorted to my unit and questioned by the officers. I didn't know this. She wanted to go and pick up our daughter but they said she couldn't leave until she provided answers. They wanted to know if I was leaving the army because of her. My discharge was put in by the Major and the psych officer, not my wife, and the reason was that if I went back to the unit I would cease to exist.

The troop commander and troop sergeant were the only people who knew that I was in a clinic – the only people from my troop who knew where I was. I hated my troop sergeant with a passion. I wanted to rip his heart out because of the things he had made me do.

When you have bipolar disorder, if you're on a high you're on a high and if you're on a low you're on a low. What this man did to me ate at me for so many years that every time I think about it, even now, I go plummeting down. Sometimes when I'm on a high something trivial or insignificant can happen and I come crashing down again. That's the hard part.

The clinic I was in simply wasn't designed for the military. The doctors kept telling me to talk to my boss as soon as I had a concern. This is highly unrealistic and unhelpful. You can't talk to your boss in the army. You say *yes sir* and do as you're told, regardless.

I did play with them a bit while I was there, I must admit. I'd tell the nurses one thing, knowing full well they were going to report it to the psych. Then I'd go and talk to the psych and tell him something else. The psych would say, 'Hey, but you said this,' and I'd say, 'Well, that serves you right for listening to the nursing staff. We're not bloody stupid, you know. We know the nurses report back to you.'

I'd get angry and tell the psych that he didn't know what was in my head. He would claim that he did, so I would challenge him. This was no help to me whatsoever.

When I was on a high I couldn't shut up. I'd tell jokes all day and get the whole clinic circled around me when I was like that. But this second time I was in the clinic I was mostly down.

I'd go out during the day and start drinking at the local bowls club. There were a couple of anorexic girls in the clinic and one night I asked them to join me down at the pub for a few drinks. When we got there, I told them I didn't have any money and the eldest one said she'd pay and I could be her toy boy. Anyway, the younger girl was pissed after one drink. I told them at the pub that we were just down from the clinic and the whole crowd literally parted around our table – getting as far away from us as possible. I preferred it that way. They left us alone.

After the younger one got drunk I thought it was time to go back. I didn't want to be the cause of any harm and we got back around dinner-time. I had ordered rissoles that night and when I went to put my fork into the rissole it literally bounced off the plate and hit the table. I picked it up and said 'Right!'

An older lady put her arm on mine and said, 'Michael, don't.'

I told her that it was my second time in here and I was sick of it. I picked up the rissole and asked to speak to the cook. I said that this was not good enough. The only thing you could use the rissole for was a hockey puck. We're not morons – we might have a mental disorder but we don't deserve to be treated like that.

Anyway I left and went back to the bowls club for another drink. I got really drunk and went back to someone's house. I didn't even know them. I just drank more and more and eventually I found my way back.

If you get back to the clinic later than 11 p.m. you have to buzz in. So I pushed the button, slurred my name and staggered in. I spent the whole night vomiting and was put on a blue alert (which means I was no longer allowed outside of nursing staff's care).

I refused to go to the counselling sessions. I just closed up.

There was one nice nurse, though. She liked my knitting. I knitted a jumper for my daughter and most people there were surprised that I could knit.

My brother had died in 1993. He had gone downhill over the last four years of his life and needed full-time care from my parents. He had a brain tumour and it had caused a lot of damage. In the end, my parents couldn't look after him any more – they hadn't had a break in four years – so they moved him into a respite home for people around his age.

Dad said my brother knew he was going to die. He wouldn't listen to the radio or read the newspaper in the end and he said goodbye to Dad. In those last four years of his life my brother tried to bury the hatchet with me, but I just couldn't.

Having my wife and daughter saved my life. They were a joy to have around.

When I look back on the things I've said and done to my daughter when I was ill – I'll never forgive myself. It's the hardest thing.

I had some semblance of care while I was in the army but after the discharge they dropped me. They refused to admit cause and I received no compensation. In 2002 I received a pension from Veteran's Affairs, who admitted that the army was responsible for the development of my disorder. I have been classified as having a medium mental disorder (no name attached).

After leaving the army, I had no set routine or medical support. The only stability I had was from my woodcarving. By this time, I was also an alcoholic.

In 1996 I decided that I wanted to be a park ranger so I began studying part time. Unfortunately, I just couldn't grasp the part in my studies about soil density, and that really got me down. At around the same time I sliced my hand while wood carving, so I couldn't do that either. I couldn't take any more. I started drinking at around noon, got drunk, then went upstairs and trashed our entire house. I can't actually remember half of the things I did, but I destroyed a cabinet that had everything from my life with my wife in it. I threw tables out of windows and smashed everything. I destroyed my daughter's room.

I was asleep on the boot of my car when the cops showed up. They told my wife that they couldn't do anything because I was asleep, but would come back later. When I woke up, I went inside and upstairs. I didn't know that I had been responsible at first. I wanted to know who had smashed the house. Then I realised and took off. I was gone by the time the cops came back and they weren't going to bother chasing me until she told them they had to find me because I had been in the army for fifteen years. Then they chased me.

This was rock bottom so I turned myself in and asked for help.

I was sent to the psychiatric ward of the Royal Brisbane Hospital but they didn't have any beds so they put me in an abandoned section of the hospital. I was alone there until the psychiatrist came. He asked what he should do with me and I asked him to send me home. He told me that if it were up to him I would be admitted into the psychiatric ward, but no male beds were available, so I was released to my parents' house.

At this point I still refused to admit that I had a problem. My wife came to see my counsellor with me and I was presented with an ultimatum – give up the alcohol or the family. Giving up the alcohol was the hardest thing I've ever done, but it's been twelve years and I haven't looked back.

Routine is the most important thing for me. If I have no routine I'm screwed. I always list the things I'm going to do the next day. Without direction, I come crashing down.

When all of this was happening, I was living on Mars bars and Cokes. I lost weight and got down to 59kg. When I went to see the doctor, he asked if I threw up when I ate anything and I said that I did. He told me that this was the beginning of anorexia and I was either to start eating now or be fed a fluid diet through a tube in my nostril. I was surprised. I began to realise that I had been trying to harm myself. I was trying to die – slowly.

To stay well these days, I focus on the positive things in life, my wife and daughter. We are a very close family. Even though my daughter is now 21, she still lives at home with us. My wife and I don't work so we get to see a lot of her and of each other. Even if we are doing separate things we are still all here together. We don't fight. I think the last time I fought with my wife was when I was still drinking, and that was over a decade ago.

I find that meditation really helps me. I don't use it all the time – it's hard to keep constantly motivated – but when I do use it, it helps.

I go to a darts club. It is a bit of a challenge for me and I enjoy the bit of socialising. I don't like getting caught up in the politics of such social gatherings but darts is something I'm good at and it's nice to get out of the routine for a bit.

My relationship with my dad has improved since he has started seeing a psych. I have been able to open up to him a bit more and I have discussed my childhood experiences with him. I told him that I don't blame him for my upbringing but just wanted him to know. Dad already knew.

Riding my bike (90 Boulevard 1500cc) and woodwork are now my favourite things to do. I carve out walking sticks and have had a number of people ask me to make them one especially. People have told me that they are beautiful.

I recently went on a long bike riding tour around Queensland with my dad. I had a wonderful time. I feel at peace when I'm riding – especially across country. City riding is still good but it's nice to get out into the open spaces. I find riding to be very freeing: I don't feel enclosed, right from the moment I put my leg over the saddle. I felt really balanced while I was on this trip.

Aside from this, my family is my enjoyment. I like my life for the most part – but there is always the potential to fall down again.

I've found that since I stopped drinking my symptoms have gotten less severe. When I was on a high and drinking I would go out and spend money just like that, but now, even when I'm high, I can still think it through rationally. My drinking was a way to escape reality but it was a bad way of doing it. It was self-medicating with bad medication. It took me further down and made me suicidal. It is really bad for your health.

You need good medicine, such as meditation. I believe that meditation is a medication: it helps but you have to do it in a good space. If you do it in a bad space it can be pretty bad. If you go in good you'll come out good.

I am now a very spiritual man. I don't believe there is a God but I do believe there is a divine being somewhere out there that is bigger than all of us.

My advice to others is to take each stage as it comes and find a good positive to focus on. You need to keep in focus whatever dream or want you have and keep it alive.

You can do it.

Ten: Lisa*

It has been a real challenge to overcome my bipolar demons.

Friends I have made since my recovery wonder at how things could have been so bad for the healthy, intelligent woman they know me to be. They ask, 'How did you go from all that tragedy to this?' It still requires daily vigilance on my part, but the self-awareness I have gained from climbing back out of that dark hole has been well worth the effort.

In a way I feel quite blessed to have had these experiences, as scary as they have been at times. If everyone took the time and effort to learn about how best to maintain their mental health, our world would be a much better place. I hope the fact that I did survive will inspire others who might not believe that there can be a light at the end of the dark tunnel of mental illness. I still have my bad days but I know why they happen and what to do about them: I don't beat myself up about being a bit more sensitive than the average human.

I was diagnosed with bipolar disorder when I was nineteen years old. At the time I had never even heard the word *bipolar* and didn't know why my college guidance counsellor had referred me to a psychiatrist in the first place. I was a gifted student at the time, excelling in English literature. I took great pride in producing consistently insightful A-grade papers but the price I paid for those

---

* Lisa Mora is the author of *I am Lisa; I am not Bipolar* (Estee Media, 2006) and describes this text as the story of her downfall. She intends to follow this with a new book, *How I Got Back Up*.

results was considerable. In order to stay on top of my studies, and to justify the exorbitant fees my father was paying, I put enormous pressure on myself.

Not yet aware of the dramatic effects of a disruption in sleep patterns on my sensitive brain chemistry, I would stay up until the early hours of the morning studying and writing assignments, often racing off to morning classes without having slept at all. This went on for months. As due dates loomed and all-nighters became essential to complete assignments or to study for exams, the pressure to maintain my thus-far brilliant grade point average increased. I eventually turned to cocaine, to stay awake and focused when I should have been sleeping. The less sleep I got the less I seemed to need, and before long I was introduced to the bipolar state that I call *overdrive*. My guidance counsellor referred me to a psychiatrist who said I was suffering from a manic episode of bipolar disorder, and prescribed Lithium.

I called my dad in tears. 'They say I have bipolar. They have prescribed Lithium. What should I do?'

'Don't take it, love,' he said. 'It will make you crazy.'

The psychiatrist introduced me to another girl at my college with bipolar disorder and she also warned me about the effects of medication. She said the pills would make me fat so I didn't take them. I dismissed the diagnosis, refused the offer of ongoing psychiatric care and soldiered on.

Three years later, after the birth of my daughter, I noticed a distinct change in my sense of wellbeing. I was constantly tired, and often snappy and irritable. This continued for a couple of years. I eventually went to a naturopath because my severe lack of energy made me feel physically unwell. I knew there was something wrong, but I had no idea what. I had already been to a general practitioner who had tested me for a wide range of ailments only to declare that there was nothing wrong. The naturopath found that I was deficient in a variety of nutrients and administered a course of vitamin B12 injections and supplements. I spent over two hundred dollars that I couldn't afford and at the end of it, I still felt sick.

It was a child health nurse who finally recognised the symptoms of a depressive episode. I was referred to a psychiatrist who diagnosed postnatal depression and prescribed a course of antidepressants. I asked the psychiatrist if the symptoms might be related to bipolar disorder, but was told that postnatal depression was common and that my symptoms were not likely to be bipolar.

Life returned to normal for a time, but when I again became depressed after the birth of my second child, I recognised the familiar symptoms and sought help. I was admitted to hospital to get some rest with the help of sleeping pills and antidepressants. After a month in hospital I attended a 6-week outpatients day program. In the mornings I attended classes on parenting issues and in the afternoons I learned about Cognitive Behavioural Therapy and Rational Emotive Therapy.

Through these classes I learned about how my self-talk or thoughts could directly affect my moods and they way I felt. With this information, I began the long and arduous process of changing those old tapes in my head and replacing them with more positive messages. Once again I was told that the recurrent depression was unlikely to be a symptom of underlying bipolar disorder.

When my marriage broke down in 1999, my world turned upside down. The man who had been the only consistent source of love and affection I had ever known did not love me any more. All of a sudden I found myself with two young children to care for alone, an acreage property to maintain and no reliable source of income. Things went rapidly downhill. Although initially supportive, the relationship between my ex-husband and me gradually deteriorated and eventually became abusive. He ceased paying child support and relocated to London.

My next relationship involved a man who turned out to be a known paedophile who, it became clear, was after my daughter. I noticed that my daughter's behaviour had become increasingly unmanageable and I consulted several health professionals about it. They were quick to point the finger at me and my earlier diagnosis of bipolar disorder as the likely cause of my daughter's troubles. One day my daughter found the courage to tell me what had been going on. I went to the police and the man was charged and convicted.

Not surprisingly, I became a nervous wreck. I wouldn't let my kids out of my sight and trusted no one. I saw a counsellor to help me deal with my extreme anxiety and he believed that I had all the classic symptoms of post-traumatic stress disorder. I was like a constantly wound spring, and engulfed with fear. I started seeing a psychiatrist who suggested that bipolar could indeed be the problem, and prescribed Epilium as I was still afraid of the possible weight gain from Lithium. Epilium nauseated me almost constantly and I had never known such a sense of fatigue. I felt as if I was constantly walking around in a fog!

Lacking skills and qualifications to gain a decent job, I enrolled at college to study homoeopathy full-time. My morning routine was insane. Each day I had to get two kids off to school before joining all the city commuters, attending classes all day, then rushing home to cook dinner and get homework and household chores done. It was even more difficult on medication because I was tired all the time. Once again I found myself staying up too late, as the only time I had to study and complete assignments was after the kids had gone to bed. I had no family around to support me, no close friends with kids. I had no one to turn to for help. I was often snappy and irritable, and unfortunately I took some of my frustration and anger out on my daughter.

The kids' father eventually came back from London and my nine-year-old daughter began calling on him whenever I had a 'wobbly'. She told her dad that I was crazy and asked him to come and rescue her. He and his partner would often call me on the phone and abuse me. He called me a 'victim' and said that he resented paying child support so I could 'sit on my fat ass'. Eventually the Department of Family Services became involved and came out to the house to interview me. They had no idea about bipolar disorder and were disinterested in my cries for help. I even gave them a book I had about bipolar disorder to help them understand. They took my children away.

That was a significant turning point in my life. I had never known depression to run as deep as it did once my babies were gone. I voluntarily went to hospital, was admitted and put on Lithium. I didn't care about weight gain any more. I just wanted things to go back to normal and to be able to cope with the stresses of life like everybody else.

At the depths of my despair there was nobody left whom I could tolerate for very long, and the feeling was usually mutual. So, yes, of course I have a highly developed sense of self-awareness; I have had a lot of free time to work on it!

Three years ago I was suffering so badly from the unpleasant side-effects of the medications that I had become toxic. I had recurrent daily diarrhoea and my weight kept dropping. I even went to the doctor to find out if I might have cancer, as no matter how much I ate, it all just went straight through me. They suspected irritable bowel syndrome, but all tests and scans proved inconclusive. I was sure that my mother and kids worried that I was on drugs. And I was! I was pharmaceutically medicated to the eyeballs. I was zombied out and lethargic all day, but when I wanted to sleep, I couldn't. I had vivid and terrifying nightmares almost nightly. The lack of deep sleep made me emotional, erratic and irritable. So the psychiatrist suggested I try adding an antidepressant and sleeping pills to counteract these problems. The cocktail was increasing in potency as pills were added to deal with side-effects of other pills. It all seemed quite mad to me.

One day I stood at the pharmacy counter with my prescriptions in hand, but something inside me knew that this just wasn't right. 'Would you take all this medicine?' I asked the pharmacist. 'Would you put all this toxic crap into your body every day?'

'Well, no,' she replied, 'but that's different.'

I couldn't really see how. No matter which way I looked at it, it felt wrong to me. After kicking the old habits of recreational drug consumption, the next step was a strong desire to pursue a life of optimum health and natural wellbeing. Of course I was scared – scared of going completely off the rails, of losing the plot, of ending up back in hospital; but somehow this all seemed pretty crazy too.

Vital steps to my eventual recovery followed shortly after this episode, but I recall this point as the first real step towards my own healing. I stopped taking medication. I still became upset and sometimes I got angry, but I didn't take these feelings as signs of failure. I picked myself up, brushed myself off and soldiered on.

It took me a long time, but I finally sought out the support I needed. At the suggestion of my psychiatrist, I started attending group therapy sessions. My experience in hospital made me more receptive to sharing my feelings with others who understood the pain I was experiencing and, slowly but surely, my fear and anxiety began to subside and I began to feel safe again.

In 2006 I published a book – over twenty years in the making – called *I am Lisa; I am not Bipolar,* about my downfall. Writing that book marked a significant turnaround in my life. Through that journey of self-discovery and increased awareness I began to understand what was needed to move beyond the label of 'defective'. I'll admit I am not proud of the details of my experience and at times I have seriously questioned why I put my name to such a tragedy, but I am proud of what I learned as a result of my experience – extremely proud. I have my scars and I am reminded all the time of how easy it is to slip back into those dark and scary places. I will never stop learning how to survive being me. My recovery will always be a work in progress.

Although my path to recovery began with the process of writing, the real work started after the book came out. I actively sought out whatever means were necessary to ensure my ongoing mental health. I moved out of the caravan park that had been my safe haven from the world and threw myself headlong back into society. I moved into the city to be closer to my children. I went to regular counselling, embarked on a fitness regime, found a passion for rock climbing and dedicated myself to a healthy lifestyle.

I have to be especially careful about how I express my feelings now that I am known as 'bipolar'. No more temper tantrums, no yelling at the kids, no more emotional outbursts. Even if all I do is dance like a wild thing and laugh out loud, people may look at me differently. No matter how big my feelings might be, there is a little voice in my head that constantly reminds me, 'Don't lose the plot, Lisa. Keep it together. You can do this.'

No more entitlement to the normal expressions of human emotions for fear of being seen as crazy again. Oh, the pressure to be perfect now! I may never be considered 'normal' again. And I'm OK with that. I know that real peace comes with celebrating our differences rather than fighting against them.

Many of my ideas about what mental illness is and how it should be treated go against popular opinion. Saying what I feel needs to be said about the process of diagnosis and the medicalisation of mental states is a bit scary, but I believe I am living proof that my way worked better for me than any of the many treatments prescribed for me. I am coping well with life and feel healthier than I have in many, many years. My family notices it, my friends notice it and more importantly, I feel it.

As a light-hearted reminder of my supposed craziness, I carry a small marble inside my purse. Sometimes while rummaging for change it rolls out. 'Oops!' I say, 'I'd better not lose that one. I might need it one day. You never know when you might lose your marbles.'

It has never failed to put a smile on someone's face. I've found that being crazy can be fun. I guess others might call me eccentric, but that title sits more comfortably with me than *mental* ever did.

I have had to work extra hard to keep as healthy and sane as possible in this crazy world. Even if I doubted the value in bettering myself for my own sake at times, I never wavered in my need to do it for my kids. After years of battling for custody of my children, I have finally been brave enough to take my case to the courts.

It's a real challenge for a mother to stay sane when her children have been taken away from her. Most animals react with what would be considered quite *mental* behaviour when their young are removed. I must admit I constantly struggled to stay on top of things without them. But I never gave up hope and I was prepared to do whatever it took to be the mother I dreamed I would be and to have them back in my life for good.

I recently achieved what I consider to be a significant milestone. Assuming that I would probably need it in writing, I recently went back to see my psychiatrist of nine years for an assessment of my mental health. This is the psychiatrist who once told me that I would probably need to take medication for the rest of my life. It was he who, at the height of my craziness and my refusal to keep taking the disturbingly mind-altering medications he was prescribing, asked me: 'How many car crashes would it take before you finally wore a seatbelt?'

Now, after I have managed for over two years on absolutely no medication at all, he says that I am psychiatrically fit and healthy, and has stated in writing that I am 'managing my condition well'. He considers my bipolar disorder to be in total remission. Oh happy days!

He warns me however, that one of his patients who had been well for fifteen years suffered a relapse and was hospitalised. I believe that I know enough now about what works for me and what doesn't to keep a close watch for any warning signs. I feel very confident in my ability to monitor my own mental health, and so does he.

I have restructured my whole life in the past few years in order to accommodate my sensitivities because, at the end of the day, that's what I believe bipolar really is – extreme sensitivity to stress in all its forms: disruptions in sleep patterns, financial pressure, lack of nutrients, arguments and conflict, traffic jams, rushing for appointments – the list of potential triggers goes on.

As a result of accepting my inherent sensitivity I have learned a hell of a lot about managing my stress levels. My daily existence is a process of constant self-monitoring and adherence to strict schedules and regimes that are sometimes difficult to explain to others, but it is worth it to be free and happy. And I'm worth it!

My mum has been a great source of support since I began my healing work, but I have had to train her too. If I got upset and called her in tears, she would often say, 'Have you been taking your medication, love?' It took a long time before I could explain to her just how invalidating that always felt. If I said, 'No,' she would implore me to keep taking them. 'You know this always happens when you stop taking them,' she would say. If I answered yes, that I was taking my meds, she would then respond with sympathy and console me. 'Oh hun, everyone has bad days, you know. I think anyone in your position who had been treated that way would feel the way you do now. It doesn't mean you're crazy.' I decided that I would spend a full year living without meds or partaking in any recreational drugs to determine if that was truly the case. During that year, I avoided the possible invalidations and dutifully answered 'yes' to all of her misguided but well-meaning enquiries as to my medication.

I still believe it is part of our life purpose to never stop learning and growing and to help each other out along the way if we can. Everyone's journey is unique and I don't have all the answers, but I am always happy to share whatever helped me along the way if it helps reduce another's suffering. Sharing was one of the most important missing links in my recovery process. It was a long time coming, but when I finally found the haven I sorely needed to express my thoughts, feelings and even anger, the real healing began. I am forever thankful to the courageous and beautiful Cynthia Morton and her Emotional

Fitness Foundation group therapy program, for providing me and so many others with that much-needed opportunity.

I was lucky enough to be introduced to the Emotional Fitness Foundation, whose policy of sobriety among participants encouraged and supported me. After about a year, a lot of counselling and adherence to some key steps, the positive changes in my outlook and circumstances were obvious. Mum said she was proud of me, of how far I had come, how much better I sounded and looked and how obvious it was that whatever the doctor had been giving me was working well. And that's when I decided to come clean. I told her I had been medication-free for over a year and explained why I hadn't told her the whole truth.

The bottom line was that the healing process involved the need to feel validated in *all* my emotional expressions, as those without a mental diagnosis were entitled to be. I was tired of feeling broken and discarded. I needed to feel whole again.

Focusing too much on a person's mental illness really does undermine their sense of self in quite a dramatic way. If you are a support person or friend, try to be aware of the impact this type of approach can have on the affected person's self-esteem. Fostering feelings of inclusiveness and belonging goes a long way in treating the detrimental effects and feelings of isolation that mental illness can bring.

For a long time I was extremely lonely. Sometimes I still am. The difference now is that I value those quiet lonely times instead of fearing them. In fact, I often seek solitude. Alone-ness does not mean I am unworthy any more. Alone time to me now means that I value myself enough to look after myself in a way that has taken forty years to develop. Alone time helps me to recharge my batteries so that I can rush back out into the world in all my boundless energetic glory, proudly declaring that I am 'tapped to the source'. During my alone times I analyse every aspect of my being: my reactions, my feelings, my thoughts, my impulses, my needs. 'How could I have handled that situation better?' I ask myself. 'What would I do if that issue came up again? Am I hungry, angry, lonely or tired? Have I been taking proper care of my physical needs? Do I have too much pent-up energy that needs to be expressed? Have I had enough exercise?' I replay every scenario in my head with the aim of ensuring that I will never feel that old level of pain again. Sometimes, if I am severely depleted and down, I just sleep, for as long as it takes me to feel better. I don't worry any more about others thinking I am lazy or unmotivated. I am extremely motivated when it comes to maintaining my own mental health.

The stigma of mental illness, the feeling of being almost branded and excluded, cuts so much deeper and hurts so much more than the classified symptoms of the actual disorder. Manic episodes come and go, depression lingers then passes, all states of emotional being are transient and fleeting, but 'being bipolar' becomes a permanent feature in your life. People look at you differently when they *know*. Getting upset over something that would annoy anyone can now be seen as a sign of mental instability.

I am not anti-medication. I do, however, have a rather big issue with the power of the pharmaceutical industry, and quite a lot of animosity towards the process of large-scale medicating when more healthy alternatives are readily available. But, having said that, I do not judge anyone who needs pharmaceuticals. In fact, I still keep a box of Lithium in my bedside table – just in case.

Whether you take the pharmaceutical approach or not, there are ways to make sure you give yourself the best chance at emotional stability and wellbeing. Every case of mental illness is unique and different, and others' symptoms are unlikely to mirror mine, so the advice of a treating doctor, psychologist or qualified counsellor should always be taken first.

By all means stick to your medication long-term, but do try actively pursuing these ideals as well and see if you don't notice the difference in your quality of life. I think everyone should follow these tips, whether or not they are mentally ill.

You are the most important vehicle you will ever have the pleasure of driving and owning. Even so, be prepared that life will still suck from time to time. As Cynthia Morton used to say in our Emotional Fitness groups, those of us in recovery often think that the universe owes us all a free ride from now on in. It can come as a shock when after all your hard work and dedication to improving your own emotional wellbeing, shit still happens and things go wrong. This is not a relapse; it's life. Sometimes it's beautiful and sometimes it just sucks. Try not to take it personally.

These are the steps I took to transform my life from bipolar bedlam to self-awareness and serenity:

Sleep

Get lots of it. I don't care what the experts say; I have found that at least eight hours a night means I function well the next day. Find out what works best for you and stick to it. Restructure your work/study/ love life if necessary to maintain your personal sleep routine, and stick to it. Naps are perfectly acceptable ways of regaining lost hours. Be warned: pulling all-nighters will always lead to disaster.

Support

It is vital! Whether it is group therapy, a good counsellor, a compassionate friend or your mum, you will need to talk things through at some point. Support people need to be strong, as you will experience anger while you work through your stuff and will probably take it out on them at some point. If you are a support person and you are reading this – please don't take it personally. A catchphrase often heard in mental health circles is *Hurt people hurt people*. I call it the caged lion response. But take heart: as you heal, the need to lash out reduces considerably. One of the many benefits of group sessions is that the facilitator regulates appropriateness of expression so no one in the group is upset, and this can work very effectively. The workshops and books created by Cynthia Morton are right up there on my highly recommended list (http://www. emotionalfitness.com/).

Journaling

Writing your thoughts and fears in journals can really help clarify things, especially when there is nobody else to talk to. Writing makes you think about how you express what's on your mind and helps you become more self-aware. As well as encouraging self-reflection and forming a written account of your reality, reading back over past diaries is also a good way to reflect and commend yourself on your progress down the track.

Avoid recreational drugs

Sadly, most sufferers of mental disorders, including me, have had exposure to illicit drugs at some point in their lives. Did the drugs cause the mental illness or are mentally ill people drawn to drugs in their vain attempts to self-medicate? Chicken-or-egg discussions aside, my best advice would be to leave all mind-altering chemicals well alone.

Caffeine

I put caffeine high up there on my 'do not take' list. A highly addictive, active stimulant with effects not unlike amphetamine drugs, caffeine is bad for you. Alcohol, nicotine, caffeine and sugar are not what many would consider drugs, but all have dramatic effects on our normal sleep/wake cycles and should be approached with extreme caution. As for amphetamines, hallucinogens, tranquilisers and the like – it's your choice, but I still maintain that successful people don't do drugs.

Eat right

It's probably the biggest cliché on the planet, but we really are what we eat. I believe that the food we put in our mouths imparts an energetic imprint on our bodies that affects more than just our digestive system. I think of food as 'good energy food' or 'bad energy food'. The further away from its original state and place of creation it gets, the less positive life-enhancing energy that food contains.

Don't get me wrong, I am no macrobiotic vegan, but I do try to keep it as 'real' as possible. As I always say, it's about respecting the vessel – your amazingly efficient body machine. Good food keeps our mind and body running efficiently and increases our ability to self-heal. Try to have as many good wholesome freshly grown fruit and vegies as you can. Choose whole grains over processed goods wherever possible. As hippy-trippy as it may sound, I believe that loving your food and appreciating it will actually help your body to absorb its nutrients too. Fast food made by teenagers who'd much rather be somewhere else than standing over a sink of molecularly-restructured grease while making your chips creates bad energy food. Partake at your peril.

Exercise

Without wanting to sound like a broken record, respect the vessel! We were biologically built to be hunter-gatherers, not sitter-waiters. Our bodies were designed to have at least a few hours a day of semi-strenuous activity, necessary if we were to eat and survive. Now we sit on the couch, at our desks, in the car, at the cinema, in cafés and restaurants waiting for others to bring our food to us. I have spent a lifetime of hating exercise. I was never the 'sporty' type. I was short and chubby, had flat feet and dreaded physical education in school. I thought exercise was about running, jumping and pushing weights in gyms and, although I did all these things in a constant effort to become slim and beautiful, I was bored out of my brain and resented every minute of it. Did I lose weight? No, I did not. Eventually I just resigned myself to being more buxom than boisterous. But then I decided that exercise could actually be fun. I took up rock climbing and I also love to dance. Although nightclubs and dance parties don't hold the same appeal for me that that they once did, house-working days are a good excuse to pump up my favourite tunes and bop around the house, arms flailing and legs flying in wild abandon.

Appreciate nature

In moments of warped perspective, I like to commune one-on-one with the natural environment. It's the most *real* thing I know. Even though my healing process began there, I found it hard to live in the city. The hustle and bustle was a constant distraction to my sense of focus. It was as though I could literally feel the stress emanating from high-rise buildings and traffic jams: I often found myself fighting the need to flee from it all. I took off in my car and sought out high terrain with a beautiful view, preferably with no man-made structures in sight. A long walk in the bush, admiring the trees and birds, provided the much-needed relief and serenity I craved, even if only temporarily.

Day trips away turned into weekend getaways until the return trips became too unbearable. I now live in a small, supportive community in a rural area in the gorgeous Sunshine Coast hinterland. The need to escape has subsided, since a glance out my window provides all the natural beauty my heart desires. As a consequence I feel more at peace than I have ever felt before. Moving here was a huge leap of faith and I don't expect anyone else to take it, but even those day trips away helped.

Growing and caring for a garden can also keep you in touch with what is real, and failing that, growing flowers or vegies in pots can keep you connected with mother earth.

Despite its ups and downs and sometimes scary moments, my journey to recovery and healing has been a positive one overall, so far. I like who I am now, and I am excited about who I will become.

Do I still have bipolar disorder? Yes, I guess I do. I am often reminded that I run at a slightly different frequency to most people.

The doctors only ever talk about the potential to 'relapse'; they never talk of a cure. Proclaiming my own wellness has not been without its pitfalls. The pressure is always there to keep it all together despite life's challenges – for me, more than most, because the expectation is that I will fall again.

Despite it all, I wouldn't trade any of my experiences, even the bad ones, for anyone else's in the world. I feel peace in my soul and joy in my heart and a sense of connectedness with all things.

I hope you feel that way too.

Resources

Good mental health involves paying attention to the physical, mental, emotional, social and spiritual parts of our lives. When we experience an imbalance in these various aspects our mental and/ or physical health can suffer. Most people experience some mental health concerns during the course of their lives. Often these are short lived*.

If these concerns become troubling in nature or don't naturally resolve, I encourage you to seek help to resolve them.

If you, a friend or loved one have concerns about a mental health issue, please seek help from your local general practitioner or qualified health professional.

A list of online resources and support services are available at www.inspiredrecovery.com/

- Lifeline Australia Help Line Ph: 13 1114 (Australia only)
- Mental Health Association NSW Ph: 1300 794 991 http://www.mentalhealth.asn.au/information/fact-sheets. html
- National Depression Helpline Ph: 0800 111 757 (New Zealand only)
- National Suicide Prevention Lifeline Ph: 1 800 273 8255 (United States only)
- SANE Line Ph: 0845 767 8000 (United Kingdom only)
- National Hope Line Ph: 1 800 784 2433 (Canada only)

---

* Source: Northern Health: http://www.northernhealth.ca/Your_Health/ Programs/Mental_Health_and_Addictions/MentalHealthConcerns.asp

Definitions*

Bipolar disorder

Bipolar mood disorder is a form of depressive disorder that used to be called manic depressive illness. People with bipolar mood disorder experience extreme mood swings – from depression and sadness to elation and excitement. The mood swings tend to recur, can vary from mild to severe, and can be of different duration.

Bipolar mood disorder affects about one percent of the Australian population, and severe disorder is experienced by about one in 200 people at any given time.

Early recognition and effective early treatment is vital to the future wellbeing of people with bipolar mood disorder. With effective treatment, people can live full and productive lives.

Major depressive episode

Signs and symptoms of the depressive phase of bipolar disorder include persistent feelings of sadness, anxiety, guilt, anger, isolation, or hopelessness; disturbances in sleep and appetite; fatigue and loss of interest in usually enjoyable activities; problems concentrating; loneliness, self-loathing, apathy or indifference; depersonalisation; loss of interest in sexual activity; shyness or social anxiety; irritability; chronic pain (with or without a known cause); lack of motivation; and

---

*   Sources: Multicultural Mental Health Australia website http://www.mmha. org.au/;
SANE Australia website www.sane.org;
Mental Illness Fellowship of Australia;
Wikipedia http://en.wikipedia.org

morbid suicidal ideation. In severe cases, the individual may become psychotic, a condition also known as severe bipolar depression with psychotic features.

Manic episode

Mania is generally characterised by a distinct period of an elevated, expansive, or irritable mood state. People commonly experience an increase in energy and a decreased need for sleep. A person's speech may be pressured, with thoughts experienced as racing. Attention span is low, and a person in a manic state may be easily distracted. Judgment may become impaired and sufferers may go on spending sprees or engage in behaviour that is abnormal for them. They may indulge in substance abuse, particularly of alcohol or other depressants, cocaine or other stimulants, or sleeping pills. Their behaviour may become aggressive, intolerant or intrusive. People may feel out of control or unstoppable. They may feel they have been 'chosen', are 'on a special mission', or have other grandiose or delusional ideas. A person in a manic state can begin to experience psychosis, or a break with reality, where thinking is affected along with mood.

Hypomanic episode

Hypomania is a mild to moderate level of mania, characterised by optimism, pressure of speech and activity, and decreased need for sleep. Some people experience increased creativity while others demonstrate poor judgment and irritability. These persons generally have increased energy and tend to become more active than usual. They do not, however, have delusions or hallucinations. Hypomania may feel good to the person who experiences it. Thus, even when family and friends learn to recognise the mood swings, the individual often will deny that anything is wrong.

Mixed affective episode

In the context of bipolar disorder, a mixed state is a condition during which symptoms of mania and clinical depression occur simultaneously: these may include agitation, anxiety, aggressiveness or belligerence, confusion, fatigue, impulsiveness, insomnia, irritability, morbid and/or suicidal ideation, panic, paranoia, persecutory delusions, pressured speech, racing thoughts, restlessness and rage.

Schizophrenia

A person with schizophrenia typically experiences changes in behaviour and perception, and disordered thinking that can distort their sense of reality. This is referred to as psychosis. Schizophrenia is a mental illness with much stigma and misinformation associated with it. This often increases the distress to the person and his/her family. Schizophrenia usually first appears when people are aged between 15 and 25 years, although it can appear later in life. The prevalence of schizophrenia is about one percent in the general population. About one third of people with schizophrenia experience only one or a few brief episodes in their lives. For others, it may remain a recurrent or lifelong health condition.

The onset of illness may be rapid, with acute symptoms developing over several weeks, or it may be slow, developing over months or even years. During onset, the person often withdraws from others, gets depressed and anxious, and develops unusual ideas or extreme fears. Noticing these early signs is important for early access to treatment.

Schizoaffective disorder

Schizoaffective disorder is a disorder in which mood swings similar to those found in bipolar disorder are present together with symptoms of schizophrenia (delusions, hallucinations, disorganised speech, disorganised behaviour and negative symptoms).

To be diagnosed with schizoaffective disorder, there must also have been a period of at least two weeks of delusions or hallucinations without prominent mood symptoms.

There are two subtypes of schizoaffective disorder: 1. Schizoaffective bipolar type – where symptoms include manic episodes or manic and depressive episodes 2. Schizoaffective depressive type – where the symptoms include depressive episodes only. Distinguishing schizoaffective disorder from schizophrenia and mood disorder with psychotic features is often difficult and can only occur over a period of time.

Borderline personality disorder

Borderline personality disorder is a pervasive pattern of instability of interpersonal relationships, self-image, moods, and control over impulses. Understanding borderline personality disorder is particularly important because it can be misdiagnosed as another mental illness, particularly a mood disorder.

People with borderline personality disorder are likely to have wide mood swings; inappropriate anger or difficulty controlling anger; chronic feelings of emptiness; recurrent suicidal behaviour, gestures or threats or self-harming behaviour; impulsive and self-destructive behaviour; a pattern of unstable relationships, persistent unstable self-image or sense of self, fear of abandonment, periods of paranoia and loss of contact with reality.

www.ingramcontent.com/pod-product-compliance
Lightning Source LLC
Chambersburg PA
CBHW070755290326
41931CB00011BA/2027

9 7 8 1 9 2 1 6 6 5 0 1 1